The 42-Da Reset

Your Personal Protocol to Empty Your Bucket and Master MCAS Naturally - Including Emergency Plans, Trigger Tracking, and Real Recovery Stories

Yvonne Cindy Searle

First Edition: 2025

ISBN: 978-1-7642608-1-7

The information contained in this book is provided for educational and informational purposes only and is not intended as medical advice. The content is not intended to be a substitute for professional medical advice, diagnosis, or treatment. Always seek the advice of your physician or other qualified health provider with any questions you may have regarding a medical condition. Never disregard professional medical advice or delay in seeking it because of something you have read in this book.

The author and publisher specifically disclaim any and all liability arising directly or indirectly from the use or application of any information contained in this book. The information provided is not intended to diagnose, treat, cure, or prevent any disease. Individual results may vary.

The protocols, treatments, and remedies described in this book should not be undertaken without first consulting with a qualified healthcare professional. Mast Cell Activation Syndrome (MCAS) and histamine intolerance are complex conditions requiring individualized medical care. What works for one person may not work for another and could potentially cause adverse reactions.

Table of Contents

Chapter 1: Meet Your Mast Cells

Your body is running a 24/7 security operation, and mast cells are the guards stationed at every entrance. They're sitting in your skin, lining your gut, hanging out in your lungs, and patrolling pretty much everywhere that connects your inside world to the outside. These tiny cells, shaped like water balloons packed with chemical weapons, have one job: protect you from invaders.

Think of mast cells as really dedicated security guards who take their job way too seriously. You know the type - the ones who check every ID three times and call for backup when someone sneezes. In healthy people, these guards do exactly what they're supposed to do. They spot real threats like bacteria, viruses, or actual allergens, and they sound the alarm. But in some folks, these guards start seeing threats everywhere. A change in temperature? Sound the alarm! Stress from a work deadline? Battle stations! That tomato you just ate? Call in the SWAT team!

When mast cells get triggered, they don't mess around. They literally explode like tiny grenades, releasing over 200 different chemicals into your body (Theoharides et al., 2012). The most famous of these chemicals is histamine - you've probably heard of it because of antihistamines like Benadryl. But histamine is just one player in a much bigger orchestra of chaos.

The Chemical Cocktail Your Mast Cells Are Mixing

Let me break down what's actually in those cellular grenades. First up, you've got histamine, which causes most of the symptoms you'd recognize as allergic reactions - itching, swelling, flushing, and that awful runny nose. Then there's tryptase, which is like histamine's less famous cousin. Doctors

1

often test for this one because it hangs around in your blood longer than histamine (Valent et al., 2012).

But wait, there's more. Your mast cells also release prostaglandins (these cause pain and inflammation), leukotrienes (hello, breathing problems), and various cytokines (these are like text messages that tell other immune cells to join the party). Some mast cells even release heparin, which affects blood clotting. No wonder mast cell problems can make you feel like your whole body is going haywire - because it kind of is.

Here's where things get interesting. In a normal person, mast cells need a really good reason to degranulate (that's the fancy word for exploding and releasing all their chemicals). Usually, this happens when an antibody called IgE attaches to the mast cell and then encounters its specific allergen. It's like a lock and key system - very specific, very controlled.

But some people's mast cells? They're like guards who've had way too much coffee and start seeing threats in shadows. They might degranulate because you got too hot, too cold, exercised, got stressed, or ate something that wasn't even a true allergen. Sometimes they go off for no apparent reason at all. That's when you might be dealing with mast cell activation syndrome, which we'll get into in the next chapter.

Where These Troublemakers Live

Mast cells aren't floating around in your bloodstream like other immune cells. They're tissue residents - they pick a spot and settle down. You'll find the highest concentrations in places where your body meets the outside world: your skin, the lining of your gut, your respiratory tract, and around blood vessels (Krystel-Whittemore et al., 2016).

This location thing is important because it explains why mast cell problems can affect so many different parts of your body.

Got mast cells acting up in your skin? Hello, hives and flushing. Problems in your gut? Welcome to cramping, diarrhea, and nausea. Issues in your respiratory tract? Enjoy the wheezing and shortness of breath. And those mast cells hanging around blood vessels? They can cause your blood pressure to tank or your heart to race.

The Good, The Bad, and The Overreactive

Now, before we start hating on mast cells, let's remember they evolved for good reasons. They're part of your innate immune system - the ancient, first-line defense that doesn't need prior exposure to recognize threats. They help with wound healing, fighting off parasites, and dealing with certain bacteria (Abraham & St John, 2010). The problem isn't that you have mast cells; it's when they become hypervigilant.

Think about it this way: A good security system alerts you when someone's breaking into your house. An overactive security system goes off when a leaf blows past the sensor. That's essentially what's happening when mast cells become too reactive. They're still trying to protect you, but their threat assessment is completely off.

Why Some People's Mast Cells Go Rogue

So why do some people end up with these overzealous cellular security guards? The truth is, we're still figuring that out. Some folks seem to be genetically predisposed - they might have mutations that make their mast cells more trigger-happy (Lyons, 2018). Others develop mast cell problems after infections, extreme stress, or other immune system challenges. It's like their mast cells got stuck in high-alert mode and forgot how to calm down.

There's also growing evidence that modern life might be making things worse. Our ancestors' mast cells dealt with actual

3

parasites and infections. Now? They're confronted with processed foods, air pollution, chronic stress, and a thousand synthetic chemicals. Some researchers think our mast cells are basically having an identity crisis in the modern world (Theoharides & Kavalioti, 2018).

The Histamine Connection

Since we're talking about mast cells, we need to talk about histamine. This chemical messenger doesn't just come from mast cells - it's also in certain foods, produced by bacteria in your gut, and released by other types of cells. Your body normally breaks down histamine using enzymes, mainly diamine oxidase (DAO) and histamine N-methyltransferase (HNMT).

But here's the kicker: some people don't make enough of these enzymes. Others have mast cells that release so much histamine that their enzymes can't keep up. It's like trying to bail out a boat with a teaspoon while someone's pouring in water with a bucket. The result? Histamine builds up in your system, causing symptoms that look a lot like allergic reactions but aren't quite the same thing.

When Good Cells Do Bad Things

Let me tell you about Sarah (not her real name, but her story is typical). She was a healthy 35-year-old teacher who suddenly started having weird reactions. First, it was flushing after a glass of wine. Then she noticed certain foods made her itchy. Exercise started triggering hives. Within a year, she was having daily symptoms that seemed completely random - racing heart, stomach cramps, brain fog, and episodes where she felt like she might pass out.

Sarah saw allergist after allergist. Her IgE tests for specific allergies came back negative. She wasn't allergic to anything in the traditional sense, but her body was acting like everything was an allergen. It took three years and countless doctors before someone finally said the words "mast cell activation syndrome." Her mast cells weren't responding to specific allergens - they were just responding. Period.

The Cellular Hair Trigger

Understanding mast cell triggers is like trying to understand why some people are jumpy and others are calm. In people with overactive mast cells, the threshold for activation is set way too low. Normal body processes - like digestion, temperature regulation, or stress responses - can trip the alarm.

Common triggers include heat (hot showers, summer weather), cold (air conditioning, winter weather), pressure on the skin (tight clothes, medical procedures), vibration, exercise, stress (both physical and emotional), certain medications, alcohol, and specific foods. Some women notice their symptoms flare with their menstrual cycle, thanks to the interaction between hormones and mast cells .

The frustrating part? Triggers can be inconsistent. You might react to tomatoes on Tuesday but be fine with them on Friday. This unpredictability makes people feel crazy, but it's actually typical for mast cell disorders. Your cellular security guards' alertness level varies based on dozens of factors - how much histamine is already in your system, your stress level, what else you've eaten, how well you slept, and probably the phase of the moon (okay, not really, but it can feel that random).

Building Your Mast Cell Knowledge

Understanding your mast cells is the first step in figuring out why your body might be overreacting to, well, everything. These cells aren't your enemy - they're more like overprotective friends who need to learn to chill out. The good news is that once you understand what's happening at the cellular level, you can start making sense of your symptoms.

You're not imagining things. You're not crazy. You're not making it up for attention. Your mast cells are just really, really enthusiastic about their job. And while we can't fire them (we actually need them!), we can learn to work with them better.

The Road Ahead

Living with overactive mast cells is like having a smoke detector that goes off when you make toast. You could remove the batteries, but then you'd have no warning for real fires. Instead, you need to figure out how to make toast without setting it off, and maybe invest in a better smoke detector that can tell the difference between burning buildings and burnt bread.

In the chapters ahead, we'll explore what happens when these cellular security guards go from protective to problematic. We'll look at how to identify mast cell activation syndrome, figure out your triggers, and most importantly, find ways to calm things down. Because while you can't fire your mast cells, you can definitely retrain them.

Key Takeaways

- Mast cells are immune system guards stationed throughout your body, especially where you interface with the outside world
- When triggered, they release over 200 chemicals including histamine, causing various symptoms
- In some people, these cells become overreactive, responding to normal stimuli as if they were threats
- Triggers can include temperature changes, stress, foods, exercise, and medications - and they can be maddeningly inconsistent

- Understanding mast cells is the first step to managing their overreactions
- You're not crazy - your cellular security system just needs some retraining

Chapter 2: What is Mast Cell Activation Syndrome?

So your mast cells are acting like overzealous security guards. But when does an overenthusiastic immune response cross the line into an actual medical condition? That's where Mast Cell Activation Syndrome (MCAS) comes in. And let me tell you, getting to this diagnosis can feel like solving a mystery where the clues keep changing and the suspect has multiple personalities.

MCAS is what happens when your mast cells repeatedly release their chemical cocktails inappropriately, causing symptoms in multiple organ systems. It's not a true allergy because you're not reacting to specific allergens with IgE antibodies. Instead, your mast cells are like faulty car alarms that go off in a light breeze, during a rainfall, or sometimes for absolutely no reason at all (Afrin et al., 2016).

The condition was only formally recognized in the last couple of decades, which explains why so many people spend years getting dismissed or misdiagnosed. Before MCAS had a name, patients were often told they had anxiety, fibromyalgia, irritable bowel syndrome, or my personal favorite, "it's all in your head." Turns out, it wasn't in their heads - it was in their mast cells.

The Many Faces of MCAS

Here's what makes MCAS so tricky: it looks different in everyone. While one person might flush and get hives, another might have primarily gut symptoms. Some people get heart palpitations and anxiety, while others deal with bone pain and headaches. It's like mast cells are playing symptom roulette, and everyone gets a different combination.

Let me paint you a picture of what MCAS can look like across different body systems:

Skin Symptoms - The Visible Ones

Your skin is loaded with mast cells, so it's often where symptoms show up first. Flushing is super common - that sudden redness that makes you look like you're embarrassed or have been drinking, even when you're stone-cold sober. Some people turn red just on their chest and neck, while others light up like a Christmas tree from head to toe.

Then there are the hives (urticaria, if you want to get fancy). These raised, itchy welts can appear anywhere and might last minutes or hours. Some folks get dermatographia - literally "skin writing" - where light scratching causes raised red lines. You could write your name on your arm with a fingernail. Party trick? More like party nightmare.

Don't forget about angioedema - deeper swelling that often affects lips, eyelids, hands, or feet. Unlike regular swelling, this comes from fluid leaking out of blood vessels thanks to those mast cell mediators. It's not usually dangerous unless it affects your throat, but it's definitely not a good look for date night.

Gastrointestinal Symptoms - The Gut Punch

Your GI tract has the second-highest concentration of mast cells after your skin, so digestive symptoms are incredibly common. We're talking cramping that feels like someone's wringing out your intestines, diarrhea that strikes without warning, nausea that makes you consider becoming best friends with your bathroom, and bloating that makes you look six months pregnant.

Some people develop food intolerances that seem to change daily. Monday's safe food becomes Tuesday's trigger. The cramping can be severe enough to land you in the ER, where they run every test imaginable and find... nothing. Your intestines look perfect on scans, but they feel like they're staging a revolt (Hamilton et al., 2011).

Cardiovascular Symptoms - The Heart of the Matter

This is where things can get scary. Mast cells around blood vessels can cause your blood pressure to tank (hypotension) or your heart to race (tachycardia). Some people experience presyncope - that awful feeling like you're about to faint. Others actually do faint.

The heart palpitations can feel like your heart is trying to escape your chest. Your pulse might jump from 70 to 140 just from standing up. Some people develop POTS (Postural Orthostatic Tachycardia Syndrome) alongside MCAS - they're like terrible twins that feed off each other (Shibao et al., 2005).

Respiratory Symptoms - The Breath Thieves

Shortness of breath, wheezing, and a tight chest can make you feel like you're breathing through a straw. Some people develop a chronic cough that won't quit. Others get hoarse for no apparent reason. Your throat might feel tight even though nothing is actually swollen.

The scary part? These symptoms can mimic asthma or even anaphylaxis. But unlike regular asthma, MCAS respiratory symptoms might not respond well to typical inhalers. You need to hit the mast cells directly, not just open up the airways.

Neurological Symptoms - The Brain Drain

This is where MCAS gets really weird. Brain fog that makes you forget your own phone number. Headaches that feel different from any you've had before - sometimes migraines, sometimes pressure, sometimes just weird. Anxiety that comes out of nowhere, complete with racing thoughts and impending doom. Depression that correlates with flares.

Some people get tremors, numbness, or tingling. Others experience dizziness that isn't quite vertigo but makes the world feel unstable. Memory problems, word-finding difficulties, and concentration issues can make you feel like you're losing your mind. You're not - your mast cells are just messing with your neurotransmitters (Theoharides et al., 2015).

The Symptom Severity Scale

Not all MCAS symptoms are created equal. Think of it like a volume dial that goes from 1 to 10:

Mild (1-3): You're functional but uncomfortable. Maybe some flushing after certain foods, occasional stomach upset, mild fatigue. You can work, socialize, and live your life with minor modifications.

Moderate (4-6): Symptoms interfere with daily activities. You might miss work occasionally, cancel social plans, or spend significant time managing symptoms. Multiple organ systems are affected, but you're not in danger.

Severe (7-9): Life becomes about symptom management. Work might be impossible. Leaving the house is a calculated risk. You've probably visited the ER multiple times. Multiple severe symptoms occur daily.

Critical (10): This is anaphylaxis territory. We're talking about life-threatening reactions that require immediate medical intervention. If you're here, you need epinephrine and a call to 911, not this book.

Red Flag Symptoms - When to Panic (Appropriately)

While most MCAS symptoms are miserable but not dangerous, some require immediate medical attention:

- Severe throat swelling or difficulty swallowing
- Extreme shortness of breath or wheezing that doesn't improve
- Blood pressure drops that cause loss of consciousness
- Chest pain (always get this checked - better safe than sorry)
- Severe abdominal pain with rigidity
- Confusion or altered mental state
- Any symptom that feels life-threatening to you (trust your gut - pun intended)

The Diagnostic Dilemma

Getting diagnosed with MCAS is like trying to catch smoke with your bare hands. The symptoms come and go. The tests might be normal between flares. And many doctors haven't even heard of it. The official diagnostic criteria require (Valent et al., 2012):

1. Symptoms in two or more organ systems that recur or persist
2. Lab evidence of mast cell mediator release (elevated tryptase, histamine, or prostaglandins)
3. Improvement with mast cell stabilizing medications

Sounds simple, right? Wrong. That lab evidence is tricky to catch. Tryptase needs to be drawn within 4 hours of a reaction, ideally at 30-90 minutes. Histamine metabolites require 24-hour urine collection during a flare. Many doctors don't know this timing matters, so tests come back normal and patients get dismissed.

The Great Pretender

MCAS is often called "the great pretender" because it mimics so many other conditions. You might get diagnosed with:

- Irritable Bowel Syndrome (when it's really mast cells in your gut)
- Fibromyalgia (when it's really mast cell-mediated pain)
- Anxiety disorder (when it's really mast cell-triggered neuropsychiatric symptoms)
- Chronic fatigue syndrome (when it's really mast cell inflammatory mediators)
- Multiple food allergies (when it's really mast cell reactivity)

I know someone who saw 17 different specialists over 8 years before getting diagnosed. She had a file thick enough to use as a doorstop, full of normal test results and referrals to psychiatrists. Turns out, her mast cells were the culprit all along.

Living in Symptom Soup

Let me tell you about Mark (again, not his real name, but his story is real). He was a marathon runner who suddenly couldn't jog around the block without breaking out in hives. Wine with dinner triggered flushing and rapid heartbeat. Stress at work led to severe stomach cramps and emergency bathroom visits.

His symptoms seemed random and unconnected. Allergists found no allergies. Cardiologists said his heart was perfect. Gastroenterologists diagnosed IBS but treatments didn't help. He started keeping a symptom diary that read like a medical mystery novel - "Tuesday: Hives after shower. Wednesday: Near-fainting spell in meeting. Thursday: Fine all day, then explosive diarrhea after eating leftover chicken."

The randomness made him question his sanity. How could he react to something one day but not the next? Why did symptoms hit harder during stressful weeks? Why did antihistamines help sometimes but not others? MCAS was the missing piece that made the puzzle complete.

The Bucket Theory

Think of your body's tolerance like a bucket. Every trigger adds water - a high-histamine meal, stress, poor sleep, hormone fluctuations, weather changes. When the bucket overflows, symptoms appear. This explains why reactions seem inconsistent. That tomato might be fine when your bucket's nearly empty but cause havoc when it's almost full.

This also explains why MCAS patients often do better when they address multiple triggers simultaneously. It's not enough to just avoid high-histamine foods if you're also stressed, sleep-deprived, and exposed to environmental triggers. You need to keep that bucket from overflowing by managing all the inputs.

The Gender Factor

Women are diagnosed with MCAS more often than men, and there's growing evidence that hormones play a role. Many women notice symptoms worsen during ovulation, premenstruation, or perimenopause. Estrogen can trigger mast cell degranulation, which might explain why some women develop MCAS during major hormonal shifts like pregnancy or menopause .

But here's the thing - men get MCAS too, and they're probably underdiagnosed. The stereotype of the "hysterical woman" means female patients often get dismissed as anxious, while men's symptoms might be taken more seriously but attributed to other conditions. Bottom line: mast cells don't discriminate, even if the medical system sometimes does.

MCAS Subtypes - It's Complicated

Not all MCAS is created equal. Some researchers divide it into primary (genetic mutations in mast cells), secondary (triggered by other conditions), and idiopathic (unknown cause). Most people fall into the idiopathic category, which is medical speak for "we have no clue why your mast cells are angry."

There's also discussion about whether MCAS exists on a spectrum with other mast cell disorders. Mastocytosis involves too many mast cells, while MCAS involves normal numbers of overly reactive mast cells. Some people might have features of both. Others might have hereditary alpha-tryptasemia, a genetic condition that predisposes to mast cell issues (Lyons et al., 2018).

The Hope Factor

Here's the good news buried in all this complexity: MCAS is treatable. Not curable (yet), but definitely manageable. Unlike some chronic conditions that progressively worsen, MCAS can improve dramatically with the right approach. I've seen people go from housebound to hiking mountains, from eating five foods to enjoying diverse meals, from constant fear to confident living.

The key is understanding that MCAS isn't just one thing - it's a syndrome, a collection of symptoms caused by misbehaving mast cells. Once you know what you're dealing with, you can start addressing it systematically instead of playing symptom whack-a-mole.

Your MCAS Action Plan Preview

Treatment isn't one-size-fits-all because MCAS isn't one-size-fits-all. But generally, the approach involves:

1. Identifying and avoiding triggers (easier said than done, but possible)

2. Medications to stabilize mast cells and block their mediators
3. Dietary modifications to reduce histamine load
4. Lifestyle changes to keep that symptom bucket from overflowing
5. Treating any underlying conditions that might be riling up your mast cells

We'll dig deep into all of these in coming chapters. For now, know that you're not alone, you're not crazy, and you're not doomed to feel this way forever.

The Validation You've Been Seeking

If you've been struggling with mysterious symptoms that seem to affect your whole body, that come and go without clear patterns, that make you feel like you're allergic to life itself - you might have found your answer. MCAS is real. Your symptoms are real. The impact on your life is real.

You deserve medical care that takes you seriously. You deserve treatment that actually helps. And you deserve to feel better than you do right now. Understanding MCAS is the first step on that journey.

Key Takeaways

- MCAS occurs when mast cells repeatedly release inflammatory mediators inappropriately, causing multi-system symptoms
- Symptoms can affect skin, GI tract, cardiovascular system, respiratory system, and nervous system - often all at once
- Severity ranges from mild discomfort to life-threatening anaphylaxis, with most people somewhere in the middle

- Diagnosis requires symptoms in 2+ organ systems, lab evidence of mast cell mediator release, and improvement with treatment
- MCAS mimics many other conditions and is often misdiagnosed for years
- The "bucket theory" explains why symptoms seem inconsistent - multiple triggers accumulate until your threshold is exceeded
- While not curable, MCAS is highly treatable with the right approach
- Your symptoms are real, valid, and deserving of proper medical attention

Chapter 3: Histamine Intolerance – A Related Puzzle

You know that friend who can't handle spicy food? Their mouth burns, eyes water, and they reach for milk like their life depends on it. Well, some of us have a similar relationship with histamine. Except instead of just avoiding hot sauce, we're playing detective with everything from aged cheese to yesterday's leftovers. And the symptoms? They're sneakier than a cat burglar at midnight.

Histamine intolerance is like having a broken garbage disposal in your biochemical kitchen. The histamine comes in through food, your gut bacteria make some more, and your mast cells contribute their share. Normally, your body's enzymes would break it all down efficiently. But when those enzymes can't keep up – or worse, aren't working properly – histamine builds up like dishes in a college dorm room sink.

Here's the kicker: histamine intolerance and MCAS often travel together like an annoying buddy comedy. You might have one, the other, or the delightful combination platter. The symptoms overlap so much that even doctors get confused. But understanding both pieces of this puzzle is crucial for getting your life back on track.

The Histamine Highway

First, let's talk about where histamine comes from. Sure, your mast cells make it, but that's just one source. Food is a major contributor – and I'm not talking about allergic reactions here. Some foods naturally contain histamine, others trigger its release, and still others block the enzymes that break it down. It's a three-way assault on your system.

Then there's your gut bacteria. Those trillions of microorganisms aren't just sitting around playing poker. Some of them produce histamine as part of their normal metabolism. In fact, certain bacterial strains are histamine-producing machines. If your gut microbiome is out of balance (and whose isn't these days?), you might be manufacturing excess histamine 24/7 (Schnedl & Enko, 2021).

The Enzyme Deficiency Nobody Talks About

Meet diamine oxidase (DAO) – your body's primary histamine-degrading enzyme. DAO hangs out in your intestinal lining, breaking down histamine from food before it can enter your bloodstream. Think of it as the bouncer at an exclusive club, keeping the riffraff (histamine) from getting inside and causing trouble.

But here's where things get interesting. Some people don't make enough DAO. Maybe it's genetic – about 1% of the population has genetic variants that affect DAO production (Maintz et al., 2011). Maybe it's acquired – gut inflammation, certain medications, or nutrient deficiencies can all suppress DAO activity. Or maybe it's both, because life likes to keep things complicated.

The other histamine-degrading enzyme, histamine-N-methyltransferase (HNMT), works inside your cells. It's like the cleanup crew that handles any histamine that sneaks past the bouncer. Genetic variants affecting HNMT are less common but can still contribute to histamine buildup.

Symptoms That Make You Feel Crazy

Histamine intolerance symptoms read like a medical grab bag. After eating high-histamine foods, you might experience:

- Headaches that feel like someone's tightening a band around your skull
- Flushing that makes you look like you've been hitting the wine (even when you haven't)
- Hives or itching that appears out of nowhere
- Nasal congestion that isn't quite allergies but isn't quite a cold
- Digestive drama including cramps, diarrhea, or nausea
- Heart palpitations that make you wonder if you should call 911
- Dizziness or vertigo that makes the room spin
- Anxiety or panic that seems to come from your gut, not your head

The timing is crucial here. Unlike food allergies that hit within minutes, histamine intolerance symptoms might not show up for hours. You eat aged cheese at lunch, feel fine, then get a splitting headache at 3 PM. This delay makes it incredibly hard to identify trigger foods without keeping detailed records.

The Genetic Lottery

Let's get into the genetic factors, because your DNA might be setting you up for histamine problems. The AOC1 gene codes for DAO production, and certain variants can reduce enzyme activity by up to 50% (Schnedl et al., 2019). It's like being born with a smaller garbage disposal – it works, just not as efficiently as everyone else's.

Testing for these genetic variants is becoming more available, though it's not yet standard practice. If you have family members with similar symptoms, unexplained food intolerances, or chronic headaches, genetics might be playing a role. But even with perfect genes, you can still develop histamine intolerance through gut damage, medications, or other factors.

There's also the MTHFR gene mutation that everyone's talking about these days. While it doesn't directly affect histamine metabolism, it can impact methylation – the process your body uses for countless functions, including breaking down histamine via HNMT. People with MTHFR variants might need extra nutritional support to keep their histamine-degrading machinery running smoothly.

The Food Minefield

High-histamine foods are everywhere, lurking in places you'd never expect. The usual suspects include:

- Aged cheeses (the older, the higher in histamine)
- Fermented foods (sauerkraut, kimchi, kombucha – basically all the "healthy" stuff)
- Cured or processed meats (goodbye, charcuterie boards)
- Alcohol, especially red wine and beer
- Vinegar and vinegar-containing foods
- Canned or preserved fish
- Leftover proteins (histamine increases as food sits)
- Certain fruits and vegetables (tomatoes, spinach, eggplant, avocados)

But wait, there's more! Some foods don't contain histamine but trigger its release from mast cells. These histamine liberators include citrus fruits, strawberries, chocolate, and certain spices. Still other foods block DAO production, including alcohol (double whammy), energy drinks, and certain teas.

The real mind-bender? Histamine levels in food aren't consistent. That piece of fish might be fine fresh but become a histamine bomb after a day in the fridge. Leftovers are particularly problematic – bacteria produce histamine as food ages, even under refrigeration.

The Bucket Theory Strikes Again

Just like with MCAS, histamine intolerance follows the bucket principle. Your body can handle a certain amount of histamine before symptoms appear. Stay under that threshold, and you're golden. Go over, and you're reaching for antihistamines and wondering what went wrong.

This explains why you might tolerate pizza on Monday but react to it on Friday. If your histamine bucket was nearly empty on Monday (low stress, good sleep, no other high-histamine foods), that pizza fits just fine. But if Friday's bucket is already full from a week of stress, poor sleep, and that aged cheese you had for lunch, the pizza makes everything overflow.

The Gut Connection

Your intestinal health plays a massive role in histamine intolerance. DAO is produced in the intestinal mucosa, so anything that damages your gut lining can reduce DAO production. We're talking about:

- Inflammatory bowel conditions (Crohn's, ulcerative colitis)
- Celiac disease or non-celiac gluten sensitivity
- Small intestinal bacterial overgrowth (SIBO)
- Leaky gut syndrome
- Chronic gastritis

It's a vicious cycle. Gut inflammation reduces DAO production, leading to histamine buildup, which causes more gut inflammation. Round and round we go, like a really unfun carousel.

Medications That Make Things Worse

Plot twist: some common medications can worsen histamine intolerance by blocking DAO or triggering histamine release. The list includes:

- NSAIDs (ibuprofen, aspirin)
- Certain antibiotics
- Antidepressants
- Blood pressure medications
- Muscle relaxants
- Narcotics

This doesn't mean you should stop taking prescribed medications! But if you've noticed increased symptoms after starting a new drug, it's worth discussing with your doctor. Sometimes there are alternatives that won't mess with your histamine metabolism.

The Testing Troubles

Diagnosing histamine intolerance is about as straightforward as assembling furniture without instructions. Blood tests for DAO levels exist but aren't widely available or standardized. Histamine levels fluctuate too much to be reliable. Genetic testing can identify variants but doesn't tell you if you currently have a problem.

The gold standard? An elimination diet followed by systematic reintroduction. It's tedious, time-consuming, and requires the patience of a saint. But it's also the most reliable way to identify your personal triggers and tolerance threshold.

Some practitioners recommend a histamine challenge test, where you consume high-histamine foods under controlled conditions and monitor symptoms. Others use questionnaires to assess the likelihood of histamine intolerance based on symptom patterns.

None of these methods are perfect, but they're better than shooting in the dark.

Living Low-Histamine

The low-histamine diet is both the primary treatment and diagnostic tool for histamine intolerance. The basic principle is simple: reduce histamine intake while supporting your body's ability to break down what does get in. The execution? That's where it gets tricky.

Fresh is best. The longer food sits, the more histamine it develops. This means:

- Buying fresh meat and fish and cooking it immediately
- Freezing portions right away if you can't eat everything
- Avoiding leftovers or eating them within 24 hours
- Choosing fresh fruits and vegetables over canned or preserved

But here's the thing – going too low-histamine can be just as problematic as eating too much. Many high-histamine foods are also highly nutritious. Fermented foods support gut health. Aged cheeses provide calcium and protein. Spinach is packed with nutrients. The goal isn't to eliminate these foods forever but to find your personal tolerance level.

The Supplement Support Squad

While diet is crucial, certain supplements can help manage histamine intolerance:

- **DAO supplements**: Taken before meals, these can help break down histamine from food
- **Vitamin C**: A natural antihistamine that also supports DAO function
- **Vitamin B6**: Essential for DAO production

- **Copper**: A cofactor for DAO (but don't overdo it)
- **Quercetin**: A flavonoid that stabilizes mast cells and may reduce histamine release
- **Probiotics**: But choose carefully – some strains produce histamine while others degrade it

The supplement game requires strategy. Taking DAO with every meal gets expensive fast. Some people save it for special occasions or potentially problematic meals. Others find that addressing nutrient deficiencies improves their natural DAO production enough to reduce the need for supplements.

The Success Stories

Let me tell you about Lisa (not her real name, but her results are real). She'd been dealing with chronic headaches, unpredictable flushing, and digestive issues for years. Doctors tested her for everything – hormones, allergies, autoimmune conditions. All normal. She'd almost accepted that feeling lousy was her new normal.

Then she stumbled across information about histamine intolerance. The symptom list read like her medical diary. She started a low-histamine diet, skeptical but desperate. Within two weeks, her daily headaches disappeared. The flushing episodes became rare. Her digestion improved dramatically.

But here's the real win – after three months of low-histamine eating and gut healing, Lisa could gradually reintroduce foods. She learned her limits (aged cheese in moderation, wine only occasionally, no leftover fish ever) and now lives largely symptom-free. She's not cured, but she's in control.

The Individual Journey

Histamine intolerance isn't a one-size-fits-all condition. Your triggers might be different from someone else's. Your threshold might be higher or lower. Your symptoms might be primarily digestive while someone else gets headaches. This individuality makes it frustrating but also empowering – once you figure out your personal pattern, you can tailor your approach accordingly.

Some people need to follow a low-histamine diet strictly. Others can be more relaxed, avoiding only their worst triggers. Some need DAO supplements regularly; others only occasionally. Some find that addressing gut health resolves their histamine intolerance entirely. There's no single "right" way to manage this condition.

Key Takeaways

- Histamine intolerance occurs when your body can't break down histamine efficiently, leading to buildup and symptoms
- DAO enzyme deficiency (genetic or acquired) is the primary cause, though HNMT variants also play a role
- Symptoms mimic allergies but are dose-dependent and often delayed, making identification challenging
- High-histamine foods, histamine liberators, and DAO blockers all contribute to the problem
- The "bucket theory" explains why tolerance varies day to day based on total histamine load
- Gut health is crucial since DAO is produced in the intestinal lining
- Diagnosis relies mainly on elimination diets and symptom tracking rather than definitive tests
- Treatment involves dietary modification, targeted supplements, and addressing underlying gut issues
- Individual tolerance varies greatly – finding your personal threshold is key to management

Chapter 4: Triggers and Flare-Ups

You're going about your day, feeling pretty good, when BAM! Out of nowhere, your face flushes, your heart races, and you're sprinting for the bathroom. What the hell just happened? Welcome to the wonderful world of mast cell triggers, where your body can declare war on you for reasons that seem completely random – until you learn to crack the code.

Triggers are like tripwires for your mast cells. Hit one, and those cellular security guards go from zero to DEFCON 1 in seconds. The frustrating part? Your triggers might be completely different from someone else's. While your friend with MCAS reacts to heat, you might be fine in a sauna but react to cold. It's like everyone's playing by different rules in the same game.

The Trigger Categories

Let's break down the main types of triggers that can set off your mast cells. Think of these as the usual suspects in your symptom mystery:

Food Triggers - The Obvious and The Sneaky

We covered high-histamine foods in the last chapter, but food triggers go beyond just histamine content. Some foods directly trigger mast cell degranulation regardless of their histamine levels. The common culprits include:

- Alcohol (the ultimate double agent – contains histamine AND triggers release)
- Spicy foods (capsaicin can activate mast cells)
- Citrus fruits (even though they're healthy, they're also histamine liberators)

27

- Shellfish (even without a true allergy)
- Eggs (particularly raw egg whites)
- Chocolate (I know, I know, life's not fair)
- Artificial additives (colors, flavors, preservatives)
- MSG and other flavor enhancers

But here's where it gets weird. Sometimes it's not the food itself but how it's prepared. Grilled or charred foods can trigger some people. Others react to foods cooked in certain oils. Some can handle a food cooked one way but not another. It's enough to make you want to live on rice and water (except some people react to rice too).

Temperature Triggers - The Goldilocks Syndrome

For many MCAS patients, temperature extremes are major triggers. This includes:

Heat triggers:

- Hot showers or baths
- Summer weather
- Exercise that raises body temperature
- Saunas or hot tubs
- Fever from illness
- Hot foods or drinks

Cold triggers:

- Cold weather
- Air conditioning
- Cold water swimming
- Ice or cold drinks
- Rapid temperature changes

Some lucky folks (and I use that term loosely) react to both extremes. They're constantly adjusting thermostats, choosing lukewarm showers, and dressing in layers like they're preparing for an Arctic expedition in the Sahara.

Physical Triggers - When Your Body Betrays You

Physical stimuli can trigger mast cells through mechanical activation. These include:

- Friction or pressure on skin (tight clothes, medical procedures)
- Vibration (power tools, riding in vehicles)
- Exercise (beyond just the temperature aspect)
- Sexual activity (yes, really)
- Surgery or medical procedures
- Massage or physical therapy

I had a patient who couldn't wear jeans because the waistband pressure triggered abdominal cramping and flushing. Another couldn't use a electric toothbrush because the vibration made her lips swell. Your body basically becomes a drama queen about normal physical sensations.

Chemical Triggers - The Invisible Enemies

Modern life is full of chemicals that can trigger mast cells:

- Fragrances (perfume, cologne, scented products)
- Cleaning products
- Cigarette smoke
- Car exhaust
- New furniture or carpet (off-gassing)
- Pesticides and herbicides
- Chlorine in pools
- Personal care products

The frustrating part? You can't always control exposure to these. You might be fine at home but react to someone's perfume at work. Or the newly renovated office space that smells "fresh" to everyone else makes you sick.

Stress Triggers - The Mind-Body Connection

Stress isn't just in your head – it directly affects mast cells. Types of stress that can trigger reactions include:

- Emotional stress (work deadlines, relationship issues, financial worry)
- Physical stress (illness, injury, lack of sleep)
- Mental stress (decision fatigue, overstimulation, cognitive overload)

Stress hormones like cortisol and adrenaline can directly trigger mast cell degranulation. This creates a vicious cycle: stress triggers symptoms, symptoms cause more stress, which triggers more symptoms. It's like being stuck in a biochemical hamster wheel.

Hormonal Triggers - The Monthly Rollercoaster

For people with ovaries, hormonal fluctuations can be major triggers:

- Ovulation
- Premenstrual phase
- Menstruation
- Pregnancy
- Perimenopause and menopause
- Hormonal contraceptives (for some)

Estrogen can directly trigger mast cell degranulation, which explains why many women notice symptom patterns tied to their cycle . Some women have their worst symptoms during ovulation, others right before their period. Tracking these patterns can help predict and prepare for flares.

Medication Triggers - When Treatment Becomes Trigger

Ironically, many medications can trigger mast cell activation:

- Antibiotics (especially fluoroquinolones)
- NSAIDs (ibuprofen, aspirin)
- Opioid pain medications
- Some blood pressure medications
- Certain antidepressants
- Muscle relaxants
- Some local anesthetics

This makes medical procedures extra challenging. You need to treat an infection but antibiotics trigger symptoms. You need pain relief but NSAIDs cause reactions. Working with knowledgeable healthcare providers to find safe alternatives is crucial.

Environmental Triggers - The Seasonal Struggle

Environmental factors that can trigger mast cells include:

- Pollen (even without typical allergies)
- Mold exposure
- Weather changes (barometric pressure)
- Humidity extremes
- Strong winds
- Seasonal transitions

Some people can predict weather changes better than meteorologists based on their symptoms. That approaching storm front? Your mast cells knew about it yesterday.

Infection Triggers - The Immune System Pile-On

Any infection can trigger mast cell activation:

- Viral infections (colds, flu, COVID)
- Bacterial infections
- Fungal overgrowth
- Parasitic infections (rare but possible)

This is particularly frustrating because you're already sick, and then your mast cells decide to join the party. Some people develop MCAS after infections, suggesting that immune activation can flip a switch that doesn't turn back off.

The Trigger Tracking Detective Work

Identifying your personal triggers requires detective-level observation skills. You need to track:

- Everything you eat and drink
- Environmental exposures
- Activities and physical stressors
- Emotional state
- Weather conditions
- Menstrual cycle (if applicable)
- Medications and supplements
- Sleep quality
- Symptom timing and severity

Sound overwhelming? It is. But it's also the key to getting your life back.

Creating Your Trigger Tracking System

Old-school paper tracking works, but let's be honest – most of us are more likely to stick with digital options. Here's how to set up an effective tracking system:

The Basic Framework:

1. Date and time

2. Trigger exposure (food, environment, stress, etc.)
3. Symptom onset time
4. Symptom type and severity (rate 1-10)
5. Duration of symptoms
6. What helped (if anything)

Making It Sustainable:

- Start with tracking just one category (like food) if comprehensive tracking feels overwhelming
- Use voice memos when writing is too much
- Take photos of meals instead of writing everything down
- Set phone reminders for tracking times
- Track for 2-4 weeks, then analyze patterns

App Recommendations for Symptom Tracking

Technology can make trigger tracking much easier. Here are apps specifically useful for MCAS/histamine intolerance:

mySymptoms Food Diary (iOS/Android)

- Excellent for food and symptom correlations
- Customizable symptom list
- Shows patterns over time
- Exports data for sharing with doctors

Cara Care (iOS/Android)

- Great for digestive symptoms
- Tracks bowel movements (important but awkward data)
- Includes stress and mood tracking
- Free version is quite complete

Bearable (iOS/Android)

- More complex but complete

- Tracks symptoms, mood, medications, and factors
- Great analytics and pattern recognition
- Helpful for seeing correlations you might miss

Simplified Trackers:

- Apple Health or Google Fit (basic but built-in)
- Any habit tracking app adapted for symptoms
- Even a basic notes app with daily entries

The Pattern Recognition Game

After a few weeks of tracking, patterns start emerging. Maybe you notice:

- Symptoms always worsen 2-3 days before your period
- Exercise reactions only happen when combined with heat
- You tolerate problem foods better in the morning
- Stress + high-histamine food = guaranteed reaction
- Certain combinations are worse than individual triggers

These patterns are gold. They let you predict and prevent reactions instead of always playing catch-up.

Common Trigger Combinations

Some trigger combinations are particularly problematic:

The Perfect Storm Combo: High-histamine meal + alcohol + stress = Major flare

The Exercise Trap: Hot weather + intense exercise + dehydration = Exercise-induced anaphylaxis

The Hormonal Hit: PMS + lack of sleep + trigger foods = Misery

The Travel Trouble: Airplane pressure changes + airport fragrances + stress + restaurant food = Vacation ruined

Understanding these combinations helps you make informed choices. Maybe you can handle wine with dinner on a relaxed weekend but not during a stressful work week.

Building Your Trigger Hierarchy

Not all triggers are created equal. Through tracking, you'll discover your trigger hierarchy:

Level 1 - The Nuclear Options: Things that almost always cause severe reactions **Level 2 - The Usual Suspects:** Regular triggers that cause moderate symptoms **Level 3 - The Sometimes Triggers:** Depend on other factors **Level 4 - The Mild Annoyances:** Cause minor symptoms you can live with

This hierarchy helps with decision-making. Maybe you avoid Level 1 triggers completely, carefully manage Level 2, and don't worry too much about Level 4.

The Trigger Threshold Theory

Your trigger threshold isn't fixed – it fluctuates based on multiple factors:

- Overall histamine burden
- Stress levels
- Sleep quality
- Hormonal status
- General health
- Medication effects
- Seasonal factors

This explains why the same trigger causes different reactions at different times. Your threshold is lower when you're stressed, sleep-deprived, or fighting an infection. It might be higher when you're relaxed, well-rested, and otherwise healthy.

Practical Trigger Management

Once you've identified your triggers, you need strategies to manage them:

For Food Triggers:

- Keep safe foods always available
- Plan meals ahead when possible
- Learn to read labels like a detective
- Have backup options when eating out
- Don't be shy about dietary needs

For Environmental Triggers:

- Create a safe home environment
- Keep rescue medications handy
- Use air purifiers and filters
- Choose fragrance-free everything
- Control what you can, accept what you can't

For Stress Triggers:

- Develop stress management techniques that work for you
- Build buffer time into your schedule
- Learn to say no to additional stressors
- Practice regular relaxation
- Consider therapy for chronic stress

The Trigger Reduction Strategy

While you can't eliminate all triggers, you can reduce overall burden:

1. **Identify your non-negotiable triggers** (the ones you absolutely must avoid)
2. **Reduce exposure to moderate triggers** when possible
3. **Build resilience to mild triggers** through overall health improvement
4. **Stack the deck in your favor** by controlling what you can
5. **Accept that some exposure is inevitable** and prepare accordingly

Real-World Success Story

Let me tell you about James (fictional name, real story). He was triggered by everything – foods, fragrances, temperature changes, stress. Life felt like walking through a minefield. He started tracking religiously, using a combination of apps and voice memos.

After two months, clear patterns emerged. His worst triggers were alcohol, aged cheese, and extreme heat. But he also discovered that he could tolerate more triggers when he slept well and managed stress. He couldn't control his coworkers' perfume, but he could control his sleep schedule and stress levels.

James created a management strategy: strict avoidance of top triggers, careful management of moderate ones, and building resilience through lifestyle factors. A year later, his severe reactions dropped by 80%. He still has MCAS, but it no longer controls his life.

Your Personal Trigger Map

Creating your personal trigger map is like getting a user manual for your body. It won't be perfect, and it'll need updates as things change. But it's infinitely better than stumbling blind through life, never knowing what might set off a reaction.

Start tracking today. Use whatever method feels sustainable. Be patient – patterns take time to emerge. And know that this detective work, while tedious, is your pathway to prediction and prevention rather than constant reaction.

Key Takeaways

- Triggers can be foods, temperatures, physical stimuli, chemicals, stress, hormones, medications, environment, or infections
- Individual trigger patterns are unique – what affects others might not affect you and vice versa
- Tracking symptoms and exposures is essential for identifying your personal triggers
- Digital apps can make tracking easier and help identify patterns you might miss
- Triggers often work in combinations, creating "perfect storm" scenarios
- Your trigger threshold fluctuates based on overall health, stress, and histamine burden
- Creating a trigger hierarchy helps prioritize what to avoid versus what to manage
- Reducing overall trigger burden is more realistic than avoiding all triggers
- Understanding your triggers empowers you to predict and prevent reactions rather than always reacting

Chapter 5: Diagnosing MCAS – The Challenge

Getting diagnosed with MCAS is like trying to catch smoke with a butterfly net while blindfolded. The symptoms come and go like an unreliable friend. The tests might be normal when you feel your worst. And finding a doctor who even knows what MCAS is? That's like finding a unicorn at a medical convention.

Here's the truth nobody wants to tell you: the average person with MCAS sees 10-20 doctors over 5-10 years before getting diagnosed (Afrin, 2016). They accumulate thick medical files full of normal test results, referrals to psychiatrists, and prescriptions for anxiety medications. They're told it's "all in their head" so many times they start to believe it themselves.

But you're not crazy. The diagnostic challenges are real, and they stem from the very nature of MCAS itself. Mast cells release their mediators episodically. Blood and urine tests need precise timing. Many doctors aren't familiar with the condition. And the symptoms mimic dozens of other conditions. No wonder it's so hard to get answers.

The Official Diagnostic Criteria

Let's start with what the experts say. The international consensus criteria for MCAS diagnosis require all three of the following (Valent et al., 2012):

1. **Typical clinical symptoms** in at least two organ systems that recur or persist
2. **Laboratory evidence** of mast cell mediator release
3. **Response to mast cell-directed therapy**

Sounds straightforward, right? Wrong. Each of these criteria comes with its own set of challenges.

Criterion 1: The Symptom Circus

"Typical clinical symptoms in two organ systems" sounds simple until you realize MCAS symptoms can affect literally every part of your body. Plus, they have to be episodic or recurring, not constant. This means you need to demonstrate a pattern, not just feel crappy all the time.

The organ systems include:

- Skin (flushing, hives, itching)
- GI tract (cramping, diarrhea, nausea)
- Cardiovascular (hypotension, tachycardia, syncope)
- Respiratory (wheezing, throat swelling)
- Neurological (headache, brain fog, neuropathy)

But here's the catch – symptoms need to be "typical" of mast cell activation. What's typical? That's where doctor education comes in. Many physicians don't recognize brain fog or anxiety as mast cell symptoms. They might dismiss your flushing as rosacea or your gut issues as IBS without considering the bigger picture.

Criterion 2: The Laboratory Lottery

This is where diagnosis gets really tricky. You need laboratory evidence of mast cell mediator release, but catching it is like trying to photograph lightning. The main tests include:

Serum Tryptase:

- Normal range: less than 11.4 ng/mL
- In MCAS: Usually normal at baseline
- Need to catch it during a reaction
- Should rise by 20% + 2 ng/mL above baseline

- Must be drawn within 4 hours of symptom onset

24-Hour Urine Tests:

- N-methylhistamine (histamine metabolite)
- 11β-prostaglandin F2α (PGF2α)
- 2,3-dinor-11β-prostaglandin F2α (PGD2 metabolite)
- Leukotriene E4

Plasma Tests:

- Histamine (super unstable, rarely useful)
- Chromogranin A
- Heparin

The timing issue is crucial. If you have a reaction on Saturday but see your doctor on Tuesday, the tests will likely be normal. Even if you rush to get tested during a reaction, the samples need proper handling. Histamine degrades quickly if not kept cold. Many labs don't handle these specialized tests correctly.

Criterion 3: The Treatment Test

The third criterion – response to treatment – seems like it should be easy. Feel better on mast cell medications? Check! But it's not that simple. Response needs to be consistent and significant. Plus, many medications help multiple conditions. Antihistamines help regular allergies too. How do you prove it's specifically helping MCAS?

The Baseline Testing Challenge

Before you can show a 20% + 2 rise in tryptase, you need a baseline level. This means getting blood drawn when you feel relatively normal (if such a time exists). Then you need another draw during a significant reaction. For people with unpredictable symptoms, this is nearly impossible to coordinate.

Some doctors recommend keeping lab orders on hand so you can rush to a lab during a reaction. Sounds good in theory. In practice? Try explaining to the ER staff at 2 AM why you need specific blood tests drawn immediately and kept on ice. Most look at you like you're speaking Klingon.

Finding the Right Doctor

Not all doctors are created equal when it comes to MCAS. Here's the hierarchy of who to see:

Best Bets:

- Allergist/Immunologists with MCAS experience
- Hematologists who treat mastocytosis
- Functional medicine doctors familiar with MCAS
- Any physician willing to learn

Proceed with Caution:

- General allergists (might only know about IgE allergies)
- Rheumatologists (might focus only on autoimmune causes)
- Gastroenterologists (might diagnose IBS and stop there)

Usually Unhelpful:

- Emergency room doctors (unless you're in crisis)
- General practitioners unfamiliar with MCAS
- Specialists who refuse to look beyond their organ system

Preparing for Your Appointment

Walking into a doctor's appointment unprepared is like bringing a knife to a gunfight. You need ammunition in the form of organized information:

Document Everything:

- Symptom diary with patterns
- Photos of visible symptoms (flushing, hives)
- List of triggers you've identified
- Timeline of symptom development
- Previous test results
- Medications tried and responses

Create a One-Page Summary: Doctors are busy. They don't have time to read your novel-length medical history. Create a concise summary including:

- Main symptoms by organ system
- Frequency and severity
- Identified triggers
- What helps/what makes it worse
- Impact on daily life
- What you've already tried

The "How to Talk to Your Doctor" Script

Here's a script to help navigate the conversation:

"I've been experiencing multi-system symptoms that appear to be consistent with mast cell activation syndrome. My main symptoms include [list top 3-4]. These occur [frequency] and are triggered by [main triggers]. I've documented these patterns over [timeframe]. I understand MCAS requires specific testing during reactions. Could we discuss a diagnostic plan including baseline and reaction testing for mast cell mediators?"

If they're unfamiliar with MCAS, you might add: "I have information from recent medical literature about MCAS diagnostic criteria. Would you be willing to review it? I'm hoping we can work together to either confirm or rule out this diagnosis."

When Doctors Don't Believe You

Let's be real – you might encounter doctors who dismiss your concerns. Common dismissive responses include:

- "It's just anxiety"
- "Your tests are normal, so nothing's wrong"
- "MCAS is a fad diagnosis"
- "You're too focused on your symptoms"

If this happens, stay calm but firm. You can respond:

- "I understand my anxiety could be a symptom, but these physical symptoms came first"
- "MCAS tests are often normal between reactions. Could we plan testing during a flare?"
- "MCAS is recognized in medical literature. I can provide recent publications"
- "These symptoms significantly impact my life. I need help finding answers"

If they won't help, thank them and find another doctor. Your health is too important to waste time with providers who won't listen.

Alternative Diagnostic Approaches

Some knowledgeable physicians use alternative approaches when standard testing is inconclusive:

Clinical Diagnosis: Some doctors diagnose based on clinical presentation alone when symptoms clearly fit MCAS patterns, especially if treatment helps.

Expanded Testing:

- Additional mediator testing

- Genetic testing for hereditary alpha-tryptasemia
- Bone marrow biopsy (in specific cases)
- Provocative testing (in controlled settings)

Treatment Trials: Starting with basic mast cell stabilizing medications and monitoring response can support diagnosis.

The Differential Diagnosis Game

Part of diagnosing MCAS involves ruling out other conditions. Your doctor might test for:

- Carcinoid syndrome
- Pheochromocytoma
- Systemic mastocytosis
- Hereditary angioedema
- Autoimmune conditions
- Endocrine disorders
- True IgE-mediated allergies

Don't be frustrated by extensive testing. Ruling out other conditions is important, and sometimes you might discover additional issues alongside MCAS.

Working with Insurance

Insurance companies often haven't caught up with MCAS diagnosis. Tips for coverage:

- Use specific symptom codes rather than MCAS codes
- Document medical necessity for tests
- Appeal denials with medical literature
- Consider cash pay for specialized tests if needed
- Work with patient advocates if available

The Emotional Toll

The diagnostic journey takes an emotional toll. You might experience:

- Doubt (maybe it IS all in my head?)
- Anger (why won't anyone listen?)
- Relief (when finally getting answers)
- Grief (for time lost to illness)
- Fear (what if treatment doesn't help?)

These feelings are normal and valid. Consider joining MCAS support groups where others understand the diagnostic struggle.

Creating Your Medical Team

MCAS often requires a team approach. Your team might include:

- Primary care physician (for coordination)
- MCAS-knowledgeable specialist (for diagnosis/treatment)
- Dietitian familiar with low-histamine diets
- Mental health provider (for coping strategies)
- Pharmacist (for medication interactions)

Not everyone needs every team member, but having support makes the journey easier.

Success Story: The Power of Persistence

Sarah (fictional name, real experience) saw 14 doctors over 6 years. She was diagnosed with everything from fibromyalgia to conversion disorder. Her thick medical file contained dozens of normal test results. Doctor #15 was different. He listened to her full story, recognized the pattern, and said the magic words: "This sounds like MCAS."

He ordered baseline tryptase, gave her lab slips for reaction testing, and started her on H1/H2 blockers. When her reaction labs showed elevated prostaglandins and her symptoms improved on treatment, she finally had her diagnosis. The validation alone was healing. She wasn't crazy. She wasn't making it up. She had a real, treatable condition.

Your Diagnostic Action Plan

1. **Start documenting** symptoms, triggers, and patterns now
2. **Research doctors** in your area with MCAS experience
3. **Prepare your medical summary** and symptom documentation
4. **Get baseline testing** when possible
5. **Keep lab orders handy** for reaction testing
6. **Be persistent** but willing to change doctors if needed
7. **Consider clinical diagnosis** if testing remains elusive
8. **Join support communities** for guidance and validation

The Light at the End of the Tunnel

Getting diagnosed with MCAS is challenging, frustrating, and often demoralizing. But it's also the gateway to treatment and improvement. Every person who's been through this journey will tell you: keep going. The right doctor is out there. The tests will eventually catch a flare. The pieces will come together.

And when they do? When you finally have that diagnosis? It's not the end of your journey, but it's the beginning of getting your life back. Because once you know what you're fighting, you can develop a battle plan. And MCAS, while complex and challenging, is definitely a battle you can win.

Key Takeaways

- MCAS diagnosis requires symptoms in 2+ organ systems, lab evidence of mediator release, and response to treatment
- Laboratory testing is challenging due to timing requirements and sample handling needs
- Finding a knowledgeable doctor is crucial but often difficult
- Preparation and documentation significantly improve appointment outcomes
- Persistence is essential – the average diagnosis takes years and multiple doctors
- Alternative diagnostic approaches exist when standard testing is inconclusive
- Building a supportive medical team improves outcomes
- The emotional toll is real but support communities can help
- Diagnosis is challenging but achievable with persistence and the right approach

Chapter 6: Medical Management

Finding the right medication combo for MCAS is like being a chemist, detective, and guinea pig all rolled into one. You're mixing and matching drugs that work on different pathways, tracking what helps, and often discovering that what works for someone else might make you worse. But here's the good news: once you find your formula, life can improve dramatically.

The medication approach to MCAS isn't about taking one magic pill. It's about creating a cocktail that addresses multiple aspects of mast cell misbehavior. Think of it as building a fortress with multiple walls – if one defense fails, others are still standing. And unlike some conditions where you're stuck with medications forever, many people with MCAS can reduce or adjust their regimen once they're stable.

The Foundation: H1 Antihistamines

These are your first line of defense, the workhorses of MCAS treatment. H1 antihistamines block histamine from binding to H1 receptors throughout your body. But not all antihistamines are created equal for MCAS.

Second-generation H1 blockers are usually preferred because they cause less drowsiness:

- **Cetirizine (Zyrtec)**: Often the go-to starter. Works well but can cause drowsiness in some
- **Loratadine (Claritin)**: Less sedating but might be less effective for some
- **Fexofenadine (Allegra)**: Doesn't cross the blood-brain barrier, so minimal drowsiness

- **Levocetirizine (Xyzal)**: The active form of cetirizine, sometimes works when cetirizine doesn't

First-generation H1 blockers still have their place:

- **Diphenhydramine (Benadryl)**: The nuclear option for acute reactions
- **Hydroxyzine**: Helps with anxiety too (bonus for MCAS patients)
- **Doxepin**: Low doses can be incredibly effective for some

The dosing for MCAS often exceeds typical allergy doses. While package directions might say one pill daily, MCAS patients often need 2-4 times that amount, divided throughout the day (Molderings et al., 2011). Always work with your doctor on dosing – more isn't always better, and some people do fine on standard doses.

Starting and Titrating H1 Blockers

Here's a typical titration schedule (adjust with your doctor):

Week 1: Start with one standard dose at bedtime Week 2: Add a morning dose if tolerated Week 3: Increase to twice the standard daily dose, divided Week 4+: Gradually increase if needed, watching for side effects

Some people need to try multiple H1 blockers before finding their match. I had a patient who tried five different ones before discovering that good old Benadryl worked best – not ideal due to drowsiness, but it controlled her symptoms when nothing else would.

The Gut Guard: H2 Blockers

Your stomach is loaded with H2 receptors, which is why digestive symptoms are so common in MCAS. H2 blockers were designed for acid reduction, but they do so much more for mast cell patients.

Common H2 blockers:

- **Famotidine (Pepcid)**: The current favorite since ranitidine was pulled from the market
- **Nizatidine**: An alternative if famotidine doesn't work
- **Cimetidine (Tagamet)**: Effective but more drug interactions

Standard dosing is 20-40mg twice daily for famotidine, but MCAS patients might need higher doses. Some take it four times daily to maintain coverage. The combination of H1 and H2 blockers is synergistic – they work better together than either alone (Afrin et al., 2016).

Mast Cell Stabilizers: The Peacekeepers

While antihistamines block histamine after it's released, mast cell stabilizers prevent the release in the first place. They're like putting a lock on the door instead of mopping up after the flood.

Cromolyn Sodium (Gastrocrom) This is the gold standard mast cell stabilizer, but it's got quirks:

- Barely absorbed from the gut (which is actually good – it works locally)
- Must be taken 15-30 minutes before meals
- Comes as an ampule you mix in water
- Tastes terrible (mix with juice if allowed)
- Can cause initial worsening before improvement

Typical Cromolyn Protocol:

- Start with 1/4 ampule in water before one meal
- Increase to 1/2 ampule after a few days if tolerated
- Gradually work up to full ampule (200mg) before each meal and bedtime
- Some people need 300-400mg per dose for effect

The key with cromolyn? Patience. It can take 4-6 weeks to see full benefits. And that initial worsening? It's actually a sign it's working – your mast cells are throwing a tantrum before settling down.

Ketotifen: The Multitasker

Ketotifen is both an H1 antihistamine and mast cell stabilizer. It's like getting a two-for-one deal. Not available in the US except through compounding pharmacies, but widely used elsewhere.

Benefits:

- Stabilizes mast cells
- Blocks H1 receptors
- May help restore mast cell tolerance over time
- Can reduce need for other medications

Challenges:

- Causes significant drowsiness initially (start low!)
- Weight gain is common
- Takes 2-3 months for full effect

Ketotifen Titration:

- Start with 0.5mg at bedtime
- Increase by 0.5mg every 1-2 weeks
- Target dose is usually 2-6mg daily, divided
- The drowsiness often improves after 2-3 weeks

Leukotriene Inhibitors: The Inflammation Fighters

Leukotrienes are other inflammatory mediators released by mast cells. Blocking them can significantly help, especially with respiratory and allergic symptoms.

Montelukast (Singulair): The most common option

- Standard dose: 10mg at bedtime
- Some need 20mg or even 30mg (off-label)
- Watch for mood changes – some people experience depression or anxiety
- Can be incredibly effective for the right person

Zafirlukast (Accolate): An alternative

- Twice daily dosing
- Must be taken on empty stomach
- Fewer psychiatric side effects

The Nuclear Option: Epinephrine

For severe reactions and anaphylaxis, epinephrine is life-saving. Every MCAS patient at risk for anaphylaxis should carry an EpiPen (or similar).

Key points:

- Don't wait too long to use it
- Common dose is 0.3mg for adults
- May need repeating after 5-15 minutes
- Always call 911 after using
- Replace before expiration date

Some patients with frequent severe reactions use compounded epinephrine sublingual tablets for milder episodes. This requires close medical supervision.

Advanced Options: When Standard Treatment Isn't Enough

For refractory cases, additional options exist:

Biologics:

- **Omalizumab (Xolair)**: Anti-IgE antibody, helps some MCAS patients
- **Benralizumab**: Targets eosinophils, may help mast cells
- Very expensive, insurance coverage challenging

Other Options:

- **Imatinib**: For patients with KIT mutations
- **Aspirin therapy**: High-dose aspirin blocks prostaglandin production
- **Cannabinoids**: Some evidence for mast cell stabilization
- **Low-dose naltrexone**: May modulate immune response

Medication Interactions and Warnings

MCAS medications can interact with each other and other drugs:

Important Interactions:

- Cimetidine inhibits many drug-metabolizing enzymes
- Antihistamines can increase sedation with other CNS depressants
- H2 blockers can affect absorption of certain medications
- Montelukast can interact with psychiatric medications

Timing Considerations:

- Space H2 blockers from other medications by 2 hours when possible
- Cromolyn must be taken on empty stomach

- Some medications work better at specific times (antihistamines at night for better sleep)

Building Your Regimen: The Systematic Approach

Don't throw everything at once – you won't know what's helping or hurting. Here's a strategic approach:

1. **Start with H1 + H2 blockers**
   - Begin one, stabilize, then add the other
   - Find optimal doses before adding more
2. **Add mast cell stabilizer if needed**
   - Usually cromolyn or ketotifen
   - Allow adequate trial period (6-8 weeks)
3. **Layer in additional medications based on symptoms**
   - Montelukast for respiratory/allergic symptoms
   - Aspirin for prostaglandin-mediated symptoms
   - Others as indicated
4. **Fine-tune and adjust**
   - Some medications can be reduced once stable
   - Others might need dose increases over time
   - Regular reassessment is key

Working with Your Doctor

Your doctor needs to know:

- Complete medication list (including supplements)
- Previous medication reactions
- What's helped or hurt in the past
- Your worst symptoms and triggers
- Your goals for treatment

Be prepared for trial and error. What works miraculously for one person might do nothing (or cause problems) for another. Keep detailed notes on responses to help guide adjustments.

Rescue Medications

Besides your daily regimen, keep rescue meds handy:

- Extra antihistamines for breakthrough symptoms
- Benadryl for acute reactions
- Prednisone for severe flares (if prescribed)
- EpiPen for anaphylaxis risk
- Zofran for severe nausea

Real-World Success Story

Let me tell you about Tom (fictional name, real results). He started with cetirizine and famotidine but still had daily symptoms. Adding cromolyn helped his gut but worsened his flushing initially. His doctor switched him to fexofenadine, kept the famotidine, and slowly increased cromolyn. After three months, he added montelukast for persistent respiratory symptoms.

The process took six months of adjustments, but Tom went from daily misery to occasional mild symptoms. He learned his medication timing (cromolyn before meals, antihistamines spread throughout the day) and keeps rescue meds for triggers he can't avoid. He's not cured, but he's living instead of just surviving.

Medication Management Tips

- Use a pill organizer – brain fog makes remembering doses hard
- Set phone alarms for medication times
- Keep a medication log to track responses
- Don't adjust doses without consulting your doctor
- Report side effects promptly
- Be patient – finding the right combo takes time

Key Takeaways

- MCAS treatment requires multiple medications working together
- H1 and H2 antihistamines form the foundation of treatment
- Mast cell stabilizers prevent mediator release but take time to work
- Dosing for MCAS often exceeds standard allergy treatment doses
- Systematic approach to adding medications helps identify what works
- Medication interactions and timing matter
- Advanced options exist for refractory cases
- Finding your optimal regimen takes patience and careful tracking
- Work closely with your doctor and communicate changes

Chapter 7: Low-Histamine Diet and Nutrition

Food should be fuel, not fear. But when you have MCAS or histamine intolerance, every meal can feel like Russian roulette. Will this trigger a reaction? How much can I tolerate today? Why did the same food that was fine yesterday make me miserable today? If you're tired of playing dietary detective while hungry and frustrated, you're in the right place.

The low-histamine diet isn't just another fad. It's a therapeutic tool that can dramatically reduce symptoms for many people. But here's the thing – it's also confusing as hell. Different lists contradict each other. Foods contain varying histamine levels depending on freshness, storage, and preparation. And your individual tolerance is as unique as your fingerprint.

Understanding Histamine in Food

Histamine in food comes from three sources:

1. **Naturally occurring**: Some foods naturally contain histamine
2. **Bacterial production**: Bacteria produce histamine as food ages
3. **Histamine liberation**: Certain foods trigger your mast cells to release histamine

This triple threat means you're not just avoiding obviously aged foods. You're considering freshness, preparation methods, and your body's individual response. It's complex, but patterns emerge once you understand the principles.

The Histamine Bucket Revisited

Your daily histamine tolerance is like a bucket. Everything adds to it:

- Histamine from food
- Histamine from your gut bacteria
- Histamine released by mast cells
- Stress-induced histamine
- Environmental triggers

When the bucket overflows, symptoms appear. This explains why you might tolerate tomatoes on a calm Tuesday but react to them during a stressful Friday. Your bucket was already fuller on Friday.

High-Histamine Foods: The Main Offenders

These foods are consistently high in histamine (Maintz & Novak, 2007):

Aged/Fermented Foods:

- Aged cheeses (the longer aged, the higher the histamine)
- Fermented dairy (yogurt, kefir, buttermilk)
- Fermented vegetables (sauerkraut, kimchi)
- Fermented soy (soy sauce, miso, tempeh)
- Vinegar and vinegar-containing foods
- Alcoholic beverages (especially wine and beer)
- Kombucha and other fermented drinks

Preserved/Cured Foods:

- Cured meats (salami, pepperoni, ham)
- Smoked foods (fish, meat, cheese)
- Canned fish (tuna, sardines, anchovies)
- Fish sauce and other aged condiments

Certain Fresh Foods:

- Tomatoes and tomato products
- Spinach
- Eggplant
- Avocados (histamine increases as they ripen)
- Strawberries
- Citrus fruits (also histamine liberators)

Leftovers:

- Any protein food that's been refrigerated
- Meal-prepped foods
- Restaurant foods (you don't know how fresh it is)

Histamine Liberators: The Sneaky Triggers

These foods might be low in histamine but trigger its release:

- Alcohol (double whammy – contains AND liberates histamine)
- Bananas
- Chocolate/cocoa
- Eggs (especially whites)
- Fish (even fresh)
- Milk
- Nuts (especially walnuts and cashews)
- Papaya
- Pineapple
- Shellfish
- Strawberries
- Tomatoes (also high in histamine)
- Wheat germ
- Many artificial additives and preservatives

DAO Blockers: The Enzyme Inhibitors

These interfere with histamine breakdown:

- Alcohol (triple threat!)
- Black tea
- Energy drinks
- Green tea
- Mate tea
- Some medications

Low-Histamine Foods: Your Safe Haven

Focus on fresh, whole foods (Schnedl & Enko, 2021):

Proteins:

- Fresh meat (cooked and eaten immediately)
- Fresh chicken (not pre-packaged)
- Fresh fish (certain types, eaten immediately)
- Eggs (if tolerated – some react)

Grains:

- Rice (white often better tolerated than brown)
- Quinoa
- Millet
- Buckwheat
- Gluten-free oats (if tolerated)

Vegetables (fresh only):

- Lettuce
- Broccoli
- Cauliflower
- Brussels sprouts
- Asparagus
- Zucchini
- Cucumber
- Bell peppers
- Carrots

- Beets
- Sweet potatoes
- Winter squashes

Fruits (fresh, not overripe):

- Apples
- Pears
- Peaches
- Apricots
- Cherries
- Mango
- Persimmons
- Blueberries (most berries except strawberries)

Fats:

- Olive oil
- Coconut oil
- Ghee (if dairy tolerant)
- Fresh butter (if dairy tolerant)

The Freshness Factor

With protein foods, freshness is everything:

- Buy fresh, cook immediately
- Freeze portions immediately if not eating right away
- Thaw and cook without delays
- Don't keep leftovers more than 24 hours
- When in doubt, throw it out

I know someone who reacted to chicken that sat in her fridge for just one day but was fine with chicken cooked and eaten immediately. She now does "cook and freeze" sessions, portioning everything immediately after cooking.

Your 7-Day Low-Histamine Meal Plan

Here's a sample week to get you started. Adjust portions to your needs and swap foods based on your tolerances:

Monday:

- Breakfast: Rice porridge with blueberries and coconut milk
- Lunch: Fresh grilled chicken over lettuce with olive oil
- Snack: Apple slices
- Dinner: Baked cod with steamed broccoli and quinoa

Tuesday:

- Breakfast: Sweet potato hash with fresh ground turkey
- Lunch: Butternut squash soup (made fresh)
- Snack: Rice cakes with almond butter (if tolerated)
- Dinner: Lamb chops with roasted Brussels sprouts and millet

Wednesday:

- Breakfast: Quinoa bowl with pears and cinnamon
- Lunch: Fresh beef patty with cucumber salad
- Snack: Mango chunks
- Dinner: Baked chicken breast with asparagus and rice

Thursday:

- Breakfast: Rice cereal with rice milk and peaches
- Lunch: Turkey meatballs with zucchini noodles
- Snack: Carrot sticks with fresh herbs
- Dinner: Pan-seared fresh fish with cauliflower rice

Friday:

- Breakfast: Buckwheat pancakes with blueberry compote
- Lunch: Chicken soup with allowed vegetables
- Snack: Baked apple with cinnamon
- Dinner: Grass-fed steak with baked sweet potato

Saturday:

- Breakfast: Vegetable omelet (if eggs tolerated)
- Lunch: Fresh pork tenderloin with green salad
- Snack: Approved berries
- Dinner: Roasted chicken with root vegetables

Sunday:

- Breakfast: Millet porridge with approved fruits
- Lunch: Beef and vegetable stir-fry over rice
- Snack: Cucumber slices with salt
- Dinner: Fresh salmon with steamed vegetables

Quick Recipe Ideas

Simple Chicken and Rice:

- Season fresh chicken with salt and allowed herbs
- Bake at 375°F until cooked through
- Serve immediately over fresh-cooked rice
- Add steamed vegetables on the side

Veggie-Packed Quinoa Bowl:

- Cook quinoa in water or allowed broth
- Sauté fresh vegetables in olive oil
- Combine and season with salt and herbs
- Top with fresh-cooked protein if desired

Emergency Snack Mix:

- Combine allowed seeds and nuts (if tolerated)
- Add unsweetened coconut flakes
- Mix in dried allowed fruits (check tolerance)
- Portion into grab-and-go bags

Shopping List Essentials

Keep these on hand for quick meals:

Proteins:

- Fresh meat/poultry (buy and freeze in portions)
- Fresh fish (eat same day)
- Eggs (if tolerated)

Pantry Staples:

- White rice
- Quinoa
- Millet
- Olive oil
- Coconut oil
- Sea salt
- Allowed herbs (fresh or recently dried)
- Rice milk or coconut milk

Produce (buy fresh, use quickly):

- Lettuce
- Cucumbers
- Broccoli
- Cauliflower
- Carrots
- Sweet potatoes
- Apples
- Blueberries

Restaurant Survival Guide

Eating out with histamine intolerance requires strategy:

Before You Go:

- Check menu online
- Call ahead during slow times
- Explain you have food sensitivities (not allergies if they're not true allergies)
- Ask about preparation methods

Safe Restaurant Choices:

- Grilled fresh meat/fish (ask them to prepare simply)
- Steamed vegetables
- Plain rice or baked potato
- Simple salads with olive oil

Avoid:

- Anything marinated
- Sauces and dressings
- Aged steaks
- Seafood (unless you're certain it's fresh)
- Anything sitting in warmers

Your Wallet Card Script: "I have histamine intolerance and need very fresh foods prepared simply. Could I have [protein] grilled plain with just salt, steamed [vegetables], and [plain starch]? No sauces, marinades, or seasonings besides salt, please. Thank you for accommodating my medical diet."

Supplements for Histamine Management

Certain supplements can support your low-histamine diet:

DAO Supplements:

- Take 15-30 minutes before meals
- Helps break down histamine from food
- Brands vary in effectiveness
- Can be expensive but worth it for special occasions

Vitamin C:

- Natural antihistamine
- Supports DAO function
- 500-1000mg with meals
- Buffered forms easier on stomach

Vitamin B6:

- Cofactor for DAO production
- 25-50mg daily
- P5P form best absorbed

Quercetin:

- Mast cell stabilizer
- 500mg twice daily
- Take with bromelain for absorption
- Start low and increase gradually

Probiotics: Choose strains that don't produce histamine:

- Lactobacillus rhamnosus
- Bifidobacterium infantis
- Lactobacillus plantarum
- Avoid: Lactobacillus casei, Lactobacillus bulgaricus

The Reintroduction Process

After 4-6 weeks strict low-histamine, you can test your tolerance:

1. **Choose one food** to test
2. **Eat a small amount** with an otherwise safe meal
3. **Wait 72 hours** before trying another food
4. **Track any symptoms** carefully
5. **If no reaction**, try a larger amount
6. **If reaction occurs**, wait until symptoms clear before testing again

Common reintroduction order:

- Small amounts of cultured dairy
- One higher-histamine vegetable
- Small amounts of vinegar
- Carefully aged cheese
- Fermented vegetables
- Leftover proteins

Managing Social Situations

The social aspect of dietary restrictions is real:

- Bring a safe dish to share at gatherings
- Eat before social events
- Focus on socializing, not food
- Have a simple explanation ready
- Don't feel obligated to explain in detail
- Find restaurants that accommodate you

The Individual Journey

Maria (fictional name, real experience) was reacting to everything. Her doctor suggested a low-histamine diet. She started strict – just 10 safe foods. Within two weeks, her daily headaches disappeared. Her energy returned. Her digestive issues calmed.

After six weeks, she slowly reintroduced foods. She learned she could handle small amounts of tomatoes but not tomato sauce. Fresh mozzarella was fine, but aged parmesan caused immediate flushing. Leftovers beyond 24 hours were always problematic.

Now, two years later, Maria follows a modified low-histamine diet. She's strict when stressed or during allergy season but more relaxed when her bucket has room. She knows her limits and plans accordingly.

Troubleshooting Common Issues

"I'm reacting to everything!"

- Go super simple: 5-10 safe foods only
- Check water source and cookware
- Consider other triggers (stress, environment)
- Rule out other conditions

"I'm losing too much weight!"

- Increase portions of safe foods
- Add healthy fats (olive oil, coconut oil)
- Eat more frequently
- Consider working with a dietitian

"This is too restrictive!"

- Start with just avoiding top triggers
- Use DAO supplements for flexibility
- Focus on what you CAN eat
- Remember it's often temporary

Long-Term Success Strategies

- Batch cook and freeze immediately
- Keep emergency snacks everywhere
- Plan meals weekly
- Find your staple meals and rotate them
- Join online support groups for recipes
- Focus on healing, not just avoiding

The low-histamine diet isn't forever for most people. It's a tool to calm your system while you address root causes. Many people can liberalize their diet over time as their overall health improves.

Key Takeaways

- Low-histamine diet reduces symptoms by limiting histamine intake
- Freshness is crucial – especially for proteins
- Individual tolerance varies greatly
- Systematic reintroduction helps identify personal triggers
- Supplements can provide additional support
- Restaurant dining requires planning but is possible
- Social situations need strategies beyond food
- Most people can liberalize diet over time
- Focus on nourishment, not just restriction

Chapter 8: Lifestyle and Home Strategies

Your home should be your sanctuary, not a minefield of triggers. Your daily routine should energize you, not exhaust your already overtaxed system. But when you have MCAS, regular life can feel like an obstacle course designed by someone who really doesn't like you. The good news? With some strategic changes, you can create an environment and lifestyle that supports healing instead of hindering it.

Think of these strategies as training wheels while your system rebalances. Some you'll need forever. Others you can relax as you improve. The key is finding what moves the needle for you without making life feel like you're living in a bubble.

Stress: The Universal Trigger

If there's one thing that universally worsens MCAS, it's stress. Not because it's "all in your head" – stress hormones directly trigger mast cell degranulation. Cortisol, adrenaline, and other stress mediators are like alarm bells for your mast cells (Theoharides et al., 2012).

But here's the catch-22: having MCAS is stressful. Unpredictable reactions are stressful. Dietary restrictions are stressful. So telling someone with MCAS to "just relax" is like telling someone on fire to "just cool down."

Practical Stress Management That Actually Works

The 4-7-8 Breathing Technique: When you feel a reaction coming on or stress building:

- Exhale completely

71

- Inhale through nose for 4 counts
- Hold for 7 counts
- Exhale through mouth for 8 counts
- Repeat 3-4 times

This activates your parasympathetic nervous system, literally telling your mast cells to stand down.

The Two-Minute Reset: Set phone timers every 2 hours. When it goes off:

- Stop what you're doing
- Take 5 deep breaths
- Scan your body for tension
- Adjust posture
- Continue with your day

These micro-breaks prevent stress accumulation.

Realistic Meditation for Busy People: Forget hour-long sessions. Try:

- 5 minutes upon waking
- 5 minutes before bed
- Use apps like Insight Timer or Headspace
- Walking meditation counts
- Even dishwashing can be meditative

Temperature Management: Finding Your Goldilocks Zone

Temperature extremes trigger many MCAS patients, but complete climate control isn't realistic. Here's how to manage:

Heat Management:

- Layer clothing for quick adjustment
- Keep cooling vests or neck wraps handy

- Take lukewarm showers, not hot
- Use fans before air conditioning (AC can trigger some people)
- Drink room temperature water, not ice cold
- Exercise during cooler hours
- Keep rescue meds handy in summer

Cold Management:

- Warm up indoor spaces gradually
- Cover exposed skin in cold weather
- Use space heaters carefully (some react to heated air)
- Warm beverages help but avoid triggers
- Layer bedding for night temperature control
- Consider heated mattress pads over electric blankets

The Shower Strategy: Many react to hot showers but need warmth. Try:

- Start lukewarm and increase gradually
- Keep bathroom door cracked for air circulation
- Shorter showers reduce exposure
- End with cooler water to prevent post-shower flushing
- Pat dry gently instead of vigorous rubbing

Exercise: Moving Without Triggering

Exercise is a double-edged sword with MCAS. It's beneficial for overall health but can trigger reactions. The key is finding your sweet spot.

Start Low and Slow:

- 5-10 minute walks
- Gentle yoga
- Swimming in temperature-controlled pools
- Stationary bike on low resistance

- Tai chi or qi gong

Build Gradually:

- Increase duration before intensity
- Add 2-3 minutes weekly
- Monitor for delayed reactions (24-48 hours later)
- Back off if symptoms increase

Exercise Strategies:

- Morning exercise often better tolerated
- Avoid extreme temperatures
- Stay hydrated but not over-hydrated
- Have rescue meds accessible
- Exercise with a buddy when possible
- Stop immediately if symptoms start

Mark (fictional name, real pattern) was a former athlete devastated when exercise started triggering reactions. He started with 5-minute slow walks. After three months, he could walk 30 minutes. After six months, he added light weights. A year later, he was cycling 10 miles. Progress was slow but steady.

Environmental Controls: Creating Your Safe Haven

Your home environment significantly impacts symptoms. Small changes add up:

Air Quality:

- HEPA filters in main living spaces
- Change HVAC filters monthly
- Consider air quality monitors
- Vacuum with HEPA filter weekly
- Minimize carpet (harbors triggers)
- Open windows during low-pollen times

Fragrance-Free Living:

- Unscented laundry products
- No fabric softeners or dryer sheets
- Fragrance-free personal care
- Baking soda and vinegar for cleaning
- Ask visitors to skip perfume
- Be prepared for pushback but stay firm

The Bathroom Overhaul:

- Fragrance-free shampoo, soap, toothpaste
- Check "unscented" products (may still have masking fragrances)
- Simple ingredients are better
- Avoid antibacterial products
- Store products in closed cabinets

Bedroom Sanctuary:

- Hypoallergenic bedding
- Wash sheets weekly in hot water
- Encase mattress and pillows
- Remove or minimize bedroom carpet
- Keep humidity 40-50%
- No scented candles or plugins

Cleaning Without Triggering

Standard cleaning products are mast cell nightmares. Safe alternatives:

Basic Cleaning Arsenal:

- White vinegar (if tolerated)
- Baking soda
- Castile soap

- Hydrogen peroxide
- Microfiber cloths
- Steam cleaner for deep cleaning

Safe Cleaning Recipes:

- All-purpose: Equal parts water and vinegar
- Scrub: Baking soda paste
- Glass: Diluted vinegar
- Disinfectant: Hydrogen peroxide

Cleaning Strategies:

- Clean one room at a time
- Open windows for ventilation
- Wear gloves (pressure can trigger)
- Take breaks between rooms
- Consider hiring help for deep cleaning

Medical Setting Navigation

Medical appointments can be trigger minefields. Preparation is key:

Before Appointments:

- List all medication sensitivities
- Bring your own fragrance-free products
- Request first appointment (less fragrance buildup)
- Ask about latex-free options
- Bring written medication preferences

Your Medical Alert Card: "I have Mast Cell Activation Syndrome. I may react to:

- Contrast dyes
- Adhesives

- Latex
- Fragrances
- Certain medications Please use alternatives when possible and have epinephrine available."

Medication Considerations:

- Request preservative-free versions
- Ask about dye-free options
- Start with lower doses when possible
- Have rescue meds ready
- Don't be shy about your needs

Workplace Accommodations

Working with MCAS requires strategy and sometimes formal accommodations:

Environmental Modifications:

- Fragrance-free workspace
- Air purifier at desk
- Temperature control access
- Flexible break schedule
- Work-from-home options

Communication Strategies:

- Focus on productivity impact
- Provide medical documentation
- Suggest specific solutions
- Know your rights under ADA
- Build alliances with coworkers

Sample Accommodation Letter: "Due to my medical condition, I require the following reasonable accommodations:

1. Fragrance-free workspace policy
2. Air purifier at workstation
3. Flexible break schedule for medication
4. Option to work remotely during flares These accommodations will enable me to maintain productivity while managing my health condition."

Travel Survival Guide

Travel challenges MCAS patients, but it's not impossible:

Pre-Travel Prep:

- Research hospitals at destination
- Pack extra medications
- Bring safe foods
- Book fragrance-free rooms
- Consider driving over flying
- Travel insurance is essential

Airplane Strategies:

- Wipe down seat area
- Bring your own pillow
- Wear mask if needed
- Pre-board to settle without rushing
- Aisle seat for bathroom access
- Inform crew of medical condition

Hotel Hacks:

- Request no cleaning during stay
- Bring own bedding if needed
- Run air purifier immediately
- Check for mold in bathroom
- Keep windows cracked if possible
- Have backup hotel options

Emergency Action Plans

Hope for the best, prepare for the worst:

Create Three Plans:

1. **Mild reaction plan** (what to take, when to take it)
2. **Moderate reaction plan** (additional meds, when to seek help)
3. **Severe reaction plan** (EpiPen use, emergency contacts)

Emergency Kit Contents:

- All rescue medications
- Written emergency plan
- Medical alert identification
- Doctor contact information
- List of medications and allergies
- Insurance information
- Safe snacks and water

Share Your Plans:

- Family members
- Close friends
- Coworkers
- Anyone you spend significant time with
- Keep copies in car, purse, office

Building Your Support Network

MCAS is isolating, but you don't have to go it alone:

Online Communities:

- MCAS support groups on Facebook
- Reddit MCAS community

- Inspire MCAS forum
- Local in-person groups (rare but valuable)

Professional Support:

- Therapist familiar with chronic illness
- Registered dietitian
- Patient advocate
- Occupational therapist

Personal Support:

- Educate close family/friends
- Set boundaries kindly but firmly
- Ask for specific help
- Share wins, not just struggles

Daily Routine Optimization

Structure helps manage MCAS:

Morning Routine:

- Take medications consistently
- Gentle movement/stretching
- Stress-reduction practice
- Nutritious safe breakfast
- Review day's triggers

Evening Routine:

- Reflect on day's triggers/successes
- Prepare next day's meals
- Relaxation practice
- Consistent sleep schedule
- Cool, dark bedroom

The Long Game: Building Resilience

These lifestyle modifications aren't meant to restrict your life forever. They're tools to:

- Reduce your trigger burden
- Allow your system to calm
- Build tolerance gradually
- Improve overall health
- Regain control

Sarah (fictional name, real transformation) started with extreme sensitivities. Her world had shrunk to her bedroom. Through gradual environmental controls, stress management, and pacing, she slowly expanded her tolerance. Two years later, she travels, works part-time, and lives a modified but fulfilling life.

Adapting as You Heal

As your health improves, you can often relax some restrictions:

- Test tolerance periodically
- Reintroduce activities slowly
- Keep core supports in place
- Be prepared for setbacks
- Celebrate every victory

The goal isn't perfection – it's progress. Every small improvement in your environment and routine can lead to better days. And better days add up to a better life.

Key Takeaways

- Stress management is crucial as stress directly triggers mast cells
- Temperature extremes require management strategies, not complete avoidance

- Exercise benefits health but needs careful modification for MCAS
- Environmental controls in your home significantly impact symptom burden
- Fragrance-free living is often necessary and non-negotiable
- Medical settings require preparation and advocacy
- Workplace accommodations may be needed and are legally protected
- Travel is possible with planning and preparation
- Emergency action plans are essential for safety
- Building support networks combats isolation
- Daily routines provide structure and predictability
- Lifestyle modifications are tools for healing, not permanent restrictions

Chapter 9: The 42-Day MCAS Recovery Protocol

Six weeks. That's all I'm asking for. Not a lifetime commitment, not a complete personality overhaul, just 42 days of focused effort to get your histamine bucket under control. Think of it as a science experiment where you're both the researcher and the subject. Except instead of wearing a lab coat, you're wearing your comfiest clothes and trying not to react to your own breakfast.

This protocol isn't about perfection. It's about progress. Some days you'll feel like a wellness warrior. Other days you'll wonder why you can't just eat a damn tomato like a normal person. Both reactions are valid. What matters is that you keep showing up, keep tracking, and keep learning what your particular body needs to stop staging daily revolts.

The 42-day timeline isn't arbitrary. Research shows it takes about six weeks for mast cells to calm down once you remove major triggers (Molderings et al., 2011). It's also long enough to identify patterns but short enough to feel manageable. You can do anything for six weeks. Even eat the same five foods on repeat if that's what it takes.

Why This Protocol Works

Most people with MCAS try to change everything at once. They read about triggers, panic, eliminate 47 foods, start 12 supplements, reorganize their entire house, and then wonder why they feel worse. Your mast cells are already in rebellion – shocking them with massive changes just adds fuel to the fire.

This protocol takes a different approach. We stabilize first, then investigate, then carefully expand. It's like defusing a bomb –

you don't just start cutting random wires and hope for the best. You follow a systematic process, make one change at a time, and always have a backup plan.

Before You Start: The Pre-Protocol Prep

Don't just wake up Monday and decide to start. That's like going to war without ammunition. Spend a few days preparing:

Medical Prep:

- Get your prescriptions filled (especially rescue meds)
- Schedule any needed doctor appointments for the six weeks
- Have lab orders ready if your doctor wants testing during reactions
- Know your nearest ER and have your medical information organized

Kitchen Prep:

- Clean out triggers from easy reach (don't throw them away yet, just relocate)
- Stock up on your safe foods
- Prepare containers for batch cooking
- Get a good water filter if you don't have one

Life Prep:

- Tell key people you're doing this protocol
- Clear your calendar of optional stressful events
- Arrange backup plans for responsibilities
- Download tracking apps or get a notebook ready

Mental Prep:

- Accept that this will be boring food-wise

- Prepare for potential initial worsening
- Set realistic expectations
- Find non-food rewards for milestones

Week 1-2: Stabilization Phase

The first two weeks are about creating a calm baseline. You're giving your mast cells a vacation from constant triggering. Yes, it's restrictive. Yes, it's boring. But it's also temporary and necessary.

Day 1-3: Medication Stabilization

If you're already on H1/H2 blockers, don't change them yet. Keep taking what you're taking. If you're starting new medications:

Morning Medication Routine:

- Take H1 blocker (like cetirizine 10mg) with water
- Wait 30 minutes
- Take H2 blocker (like famotidine 20mg)
- Eat breakfast 15 minutes later

Evening Medication Routine:

- H2 blocker with dinner
- H1 blocker at bedtime
- Any prescribed mast cell stabilizers as directed

Don't expect immediate improvement. Some people feel better within days, others take weeks. A few temporarily feel worse as their bodies adjust. Track everything – time taken, any immediate reactions, overall daily symptoms.

The Stabilization Diet

For these two weeks, you're eating only the safest of safe foods. I'm talking boring. I'm talking repetitive. I'm talking about your taste buds filing a formal complaint. Too bad. They'll survive.

Your 10-15 Safe Foods List:

- White rice (fresh cooked daily)
- Sweet potatoes (baked, not fried)
- Fresh chicken breast (cooked and eaten immediately)
- Zucchini (steamed or sautéed in allowed oil)
- Carrots (cooked, not raw)
- Brussels sprouts
- Cauliflower
- Blueberries (fresh, not frozen)
- Apples (peeled)
- Olive oil
- Sea salt
- Fresh herbs like basil or oregano (if tolerated)
- Rice milk (unsweetened)
- Herbal tea (chamomile or ginger)

That's it. No cheating. No "just a bite." No "but it's organic." Your mast cells don't care about your food philosophy – they care about not being triggered.

Sample Day Menu:

- Breakfast: Rice porridge with blueberries and rice milk
- Snack: Apple slices
- Lunch: Grilled chicken with steamed carrots and zucchini
- Snack: Sweet potato rounds with sea salt
- Dinner: Chicken with cauliflower rice and Brussels sprouts
- Evening: Chamomile tea

Exciting? No. Effective? Yes.

Symptom Tracking Basics

Get a notebook or app and track:

- Everything you eat with times
- All symptoms with times and severity (1-10 scale)
- Medications taken
- Sleep quality
- Stress level
- Environmental factors (weather, exposures)

Don't overthink it. Simple is better than perfect. "2pm - ate chicken and rice. 3pm - mild headache (4/10). 4pm - headache gone." That's enough.

Stress Reduction Foundation

Stress directly triggers mast cells, so basic stress management isn't optional. For these two weeks, focus on:

Daily 4-7-8 Breathing: Do this 3x daily minimum:

- Exhale completely
- Inhale through nose for 4 counts
- Hold for 7 counts
- Exhale through mouth for 8 counts
- Repeat 4 times

The 20-Minute Walk: Every day, no excuses (unless you're reacting). Gentle pace. If outside triggers you, walk indoors. If standing triggers you, do seated movements. Adapt but don't skip.

Evening Wind-Down:

- All screens off by 9 PM
- Dim lights

- Gentle stretching or yoga
- Journaling about the day
- Gratitude practice (even if it's "grateful this day is over")

Environmental Controls

Your home needs to be your safe zone. This week, focus on your bedroom and kitchen:

Bedroom Makeover:

- Remove all fragranced items
- Wash bedding in fragrance-free detergent
- HEPA filter running 24/7
- Temperature control (cool is usually better)
- Blackout curtains for better sleep

Kitchen Clean-Up:

- Store trigger foods where you won't see them
- Clean surfaces with baking soda/water
- Check for hidden mold under sink
- Use glass containers, not plastic
- Run exhaust fan while cooking

Days 4-7: Finding Your Rhythm

By day 4, you should have a routine starting. This is when most people either feel slightly better or hit the "detox" wall. If you feel worse before better, that's actually normal. Your body is adjusting to the lack of constant triggers.

Common experiences:

- Headaches from histamine withdrawal
- Fatigue as your body recalibrates
- Mood swings from food boredom

- Digestive changes as gut bacteria adjust
- Better sleep (eventually)

Keep going. Don't add new foods yet. Don't adjust medications. Just maintain the boring stability.

Days 8-14: Stabilization Deepens

Week 2 is when patterns emerge. You might notice:

- Certain times of day are worse
- Symptoms cluster together
- Some safe foods aren't so safe
- Medications work better with specific timing

Fine-Tuning Your Safe Foods: If you're still reacting, cut back to 5-6 foods:

- White rice
- One protein (chicken or lamb)
- Two vegetables (zucchini and carrots)
- One oil (olive)
- Salt

Yes, it's extreme. It's also temporary. Once stable for 3-4 days, slowly add back the other safe foods one at a time.

Medication Timing Adjustments: Track when symptoms occur and adjust medication timing:

- Morning reactions? Take H1 blocker earlier
- Afternoon slump? Split H2 blocker doses
- Night symptoms? Add evening H1 blocker
- Work with your doctor on all adjustments

The Stabilization Checkpoint

By day 14, assess your progress:

Green Light to Proceed:

- Symptoms reduced by 30% or more
- Consistent pattern identification
- Tolerating all safe foods
- Medications helping somewhat
- Energy slightly improved

Yellow Light - Modify:

- Some improvement but still significant symptoms
- Can't tolerate all safe foods
- Medications causing side effects
- Need to simplify further

Red Light - Seek Help:

- Symptoms worsening significantly
- New severe symptoms appearing
- Unable to maintain nutrition
- Medications not helping at all

Week 3-4: Identification Phase

Now that your system has calmed down (hopefully), it's time to play detective. These two weeks are about understanding your unique triggers and patterns.

Continuing Medications

Keep taking your H1/H2 blockers but now track more precisely:

- Does taking them with food work better?
- Do you need higher doses at certain times?
- Are side effects manageable?

- Do you need dose adjustments?

If you're on mast cell stabilizers like cromolyn, you should start seeing benefits now. Don't stop if you don't feel dramatic improvement – these medications work slowly.

Advanced Food Diary Techniques

Your tracking levels up now. For each meal, note:

- Exact time eaten
- Quantity of each food
- Cooking method
- How fresh it was
- Any symptoms in next 4 hours
- Delayed symptoms (next day)
- Overall daily rating

Look for patterns:

- Do you react to larger portions?
- Is fresh-cooked better than leftovers?
- Does cooking method matter?
- Are morning foods better tolerated?

Identifying Your Top Triggers

By now, patterns should emerge. Your top 3-5 triggers might be:

Food-Related:

- Specific foods (even "safe" ones)
- Eating too much at once
- Food temperature
- Time between cooking and eating

Environmental:

- Temperature changes
- Humidity levels
- Fragrances/chemicals
- Seasonal allergens

Physical:

- Exercise intensity
- Sleep deprivation
- Tight clothing
- Physical stress

Emotional:

- Work stress
- Relationship tension
- Financial worry
- Health anxiety

Adding Gentle Movement

Exercise is tricky with MCAS. Start ridiculously easy:

Week 3 Movement:

- 5-minute gentle walk daily
- Basic stretching routine
- Deep breathing exercises
- Gentle yoga if tolerated

Week 4 Progression:

- 10-minute walks
- Light resistance bands
- Swimming if available (watch for chlorine)
- Tai chi movements

Signs you're overdoing it:

- Flushing during/after exercise
- Delayed fatigue (next day)
- Increased reactions to foods
- Heart rate staying elevated
- New symptoms appearing

Sleep Hygiene Implementation

Poor sleep worsens everything. This phase focuses on optimization:

The MCAS Sleep Protocol:

- Bedroom temperature 65-68°F
- Complete darkness (cover LED lights)
- White noise machine if helpful
- Same bedtime/wake time daily
- No eating 3 hours before bed
- Medications timed for best sleep

Pre-Sleep Routine (starts 90 minutes before bed):

- Warm (not hot) shower
- Gentle stretching
- Journaling worries out
- Progressive muscle relaxation
- Gratitude practice
- Reading (not screens)

Days 15-21: Pattern Recognition

This week is about connecting dots. Review your tracking and look for:

Timing Patterns:

- Morning vs. evening symptoms
- Reactions after specific intervals
- Weekly patterns (worse on Mondays?)
- Menstrual cycle connections

Combination Triggers:

- Food + stress = reaction
- Exercise + heat = symptoms
- Poor sleep + triggers = flare
- Multiple small triggers = big reaction

Creating Your Trigger Map

Draw or list your triggers in categories:

Always Triggers (avoid completely):

- [Your worst foods]
- [Your worst environmental triggers]
- [Your worst stressors]

Sometimes Triggers (dose-dependent):

- [Foods okay in small amounts]
- [Tolerable activities with limits]
- [Manageable stressors]

Rarely Triggers (usually safe):

- [Your safest foods]
- [Your safest environments]
- [Your coping activities]

Days 22-28: Refining Understanding

The fourth week deepens your self-knowledge:

Medication Refinement: Track if you need:

- Different doses for different triggers
- Preventive dosing before known exposures
- Rescue medications for reactions
- Timing adjustments for activities

Exercise Tolerance Testing: Carefully test your limits:

- Increase duration by 2 minutes
- Try different times of day
- Test different temperatures
- Note delayed reactions

Stress Response Patterns: Identify how stress affects you:

- Immediate reactions?
- Delayed symptoms?
- Which stressors are worst?
- What actually helps?

Week 5-6: Expansion Phase

You've stabilized. You've identified triggers. Now it's time to carefully expand your life again. This phase is about finding your personal balance between safety and quality of life.

Food Reintroduction Protocol

Add one new food every 3 days. Not 2 days. Not "close enough to 3 days." Actually 3 days. Reactions can be delayed 48-72 hours.

How to Test Foods:

Day 1 Morning:

95

- Eat small amount (2 tablespoons) of new food
- With otherwise safe meal
- Track for 4 hours

Day 1 Afternoon (if no reaction):

- Eat normal portion
- Continue tracking

Days 2-3:

- Don't eat the new food
- Watch for delayed reactions
- Track all symptoms

Day 4:

- If no reactions, add to "sometimes safe" list
- If reactions occurred, wait 2 weeks to retry
- Start next food test

Smart Reintroduction Order:

Start with foods least likely to trigger:

1. Low-histamine vegetables (lettuce, cucumbers)
2. Additional proteins (turkey, lamb)
3. More fruits (pears, mangoes)
4. Whole grains (quinoa, buckwheat)
5. Healthy fats (coconut oil, ghee if dairy tolerant)

Then moderate-risk foods: 6. Eggs (start with yolks) 7. Nuts/seeds (start with almonds) 8. Dairy (if tolerated, start with butter) 9. Legumes (white beans first)

Leave high-risk foods for last (or never):

- Fermented foods
- Aged cheeses
- Processed meats
- Alcohol
- Vinegar
- Leftover proteins

Medication Pattern Adjustments

By now you know your patterns. Work with your doctor to:

- Adjust baseline doses
- Add preventive dosing for triggers
- Optimize timing for your schedule
- Consider additional medications if needed

Example adjustment: "I need extra H1 blocker on high-pollen days and double H2 blockers when eating out. My baseline works for normal days."

Emergency Action Plan Development

Hope for the best, prepare for the worst. Create three plans:

Mild Reaction Plan:

- Take extra H1 blocker
- Use rescue antihistamine
- Remove yourself from triggers
- Rest and hydrate
- Track what happened

Moderate Reaction Plan:

- All of the above plus:
- Call someone for support
- Consider urgent care if not improving

- Use prescribed rescue medications
- Cancel activities

Severe Reaction Plan:

- Use EpiPen if prescribed
- Call 911
- Have someone drive you to ER
- Bring medication list
- Don't wait "to see if it improves"

Sustainable Meal Planning

You can't eat 10 foods forever. Build a rotation that works:

The Rule of Three:

- 3 breakfast options
- 3 lunch templates
- 3 dinner templates
- 3 safe snacks
- 3 emergency meals

Batch Cooking Strategy:

- Cook proteins immediately after shopping
- Freeze in meal portions
- Prep vegetables for 2-3 days max
- Keep emergency meals always ready

Shopping Schedule:

- Proteins: 2x per week
- Vegetables: 2-3x per week
- Safe non-perishables: monthly
- Always have backup options

Building Your Support System

You need people who get it:

Medical Team:

- Primary doctor who listens
- Specialist who knows MCAS
- Pharmacist who understands sensitivities
- Therapist for chronic illness coping

Personal Support:

- One person who really understands
- Family members who respect your needs
- Friends who accommodate restrictions
- Online community for validation

Practical Support:

- Someone to call in emergencies
- Backup for responsibilities
- Help with shopping if needed
- Meal prep assistance if helpful

Days 29-35: Integration

This week focuses on making it all sustainable:

Creating Flexibility:

- Plan for eating out (call ahead, bring safe foods)
- Travel preparations (pack medications, research hospitals)
- Work accommodations (fragrance-free space, food storage)
- Social strategies (eat before, bring safe options)

Testing Boundaries:

- Try a restaurant with safe options
- Attend a short social event
- Take a day trip
- Push one boundary at a time

Days 36-42: Your New Normal

The final week is about creating your personalized long-term plan:

What's Working:

- Which medications at what doses
- Which foods in what amounts
- Which activities with what modifications
- Which strategies for what situations

What Needs Adjustment:

- Remaining symptoms to address
- Quality of life improvements needed
- Support systems to strengthen
- Medical follow-up required

Your Daily Success Framework

Every day doesn't have to be perfect, but it should include:

Morning Routine (20 minutes):

- Take medications consistently
- Check in with your body
- Eat safe breakfast
- Review day for triggers
- Set realistic intentions

Midday Check-in (5 minutes):

- How are symptoms?
- Any unexpected triggers?
- Medication reminders
- Hydration check
- Stress level assessment

Evening Routine (15 minutes):

- Track the day
- Prep tomorrow's meals
- Evening medications
- Gentle movement
- Gratitude practice

Creating Your Personal Protocol

After 42 days, you'll have your blueprint:

Your Safe Foods: [List of 20-30 foods you tolerate]

Your Trigger List: [Organized by severity]

Your Medication Schedule: [What, when, how much]

Your Movement Plan: [Type, duration, timing]

Your Stress Management: [What actually works]

Your Emergency Protocol: [Step-by-step plans]

Your Support System: [Who to call when]

The Reality Check

This protocol isn't a cure. Some days will still suck. You'll still react to things. You'll still wish you could eat pizza without planning for war. But here's what you will have:

- Significantly fewer daily symptoms
- Predictability in your reactions
- Confidence in your management
- Tools for handling flares
- A life beyond constant reactions

Jenny (fictional name, real results) went from 8-10 daily reactions to 1-2 weekly. She can work part-time, travel carefully, and even eat at three restaurants. Not perfect, but livable.

Robert started unable to leave his house. After 42 days, he grocery shops weekly, walks daily, and has dinner with family on Sundays. He still can't do everything, but he can do enough.

Your 42-Day Commitment

This protocol asks for six weeks of serious commitment. Boring food, detailed tracking, lifestyle changes, and patience. In return, you get your life back. Not your old life – that ship has sailed. But a new life where you're in control instead of your mast cells.

Start when you're ready. Not when it's convenient (it never will be). Not when life is calm (it rarely is). Start when you're sick of feeling sick and ready to do something about it.

Six weeks. 42 days. 1,008 hours. That's all that stands between you and understanding your body well enough to work with it instead of against it. You've probably spent longer than that feeling miserable. Isn't it time to spend that time getting better?

Key Takeaways

- The 42-day protocol progresses through stabilization, identification, and expansion phases
- Week 1-2 focuses on calming your system with minimal triggers and basic medications
- Week 3-4 identifies your unique triggers and patterns through careful tracking
- Week 5-6 expands your diet and activities while building sustainable routines
- Success requires boring consistency, not perfection
- Daily routines create the framework for long-term management
- Building support systems is essential for sustainable success
- The goal is significant improvement, not cure
- Your personal protocol emerges from tracking your individual responses
- Six weeks of commitment can change your relationship with MCAS

Chapter 10: Comorbidities and Overlaps

Your body isn't running separate systems that never talk to each other. It's more like a chaotic group chat where everyone's responding to everyone else's messages, often at the same time. When you have MCAS, you're rarely dealing with just mast cells gone wild. You're usually juggling a whole circus of interconnected conditions that feed off each other like a biochemical feedback loop from hell.

The medical system loves to put conditions in neat little boxes. You see the rheumatologist for joint pain, the cardiologist for heart issues, the gastroenterologist for gut problems. But what if all these seemingly separate issues stem from the same root cause? What if your bendy joints, racing heart, and angry gut are all part of the same syndrome? That's where understanding comorbidities becomes crucial.

The Unholy Trinity: MCAS, EDS, and POTS

If MCAS had best friends, they'd be Ehlers-Danlos Syndrome (EDS) and Postural Orthostatic Tachycardia Syndrome (POTS). These three conditions show up together so often, researchers are scrambling to understand why (Cheung & Vadas, 2015).

Ehlers-Danlos Syndrome - When Everything's Too Stretchy

EDS is a connective tissue disorder where your collagen is basically defective. Think of collagen as the glue holding your body together. In EDS, that glue is more like silly putty. The result?

- Hypermobile joints that bend way too far
- Skin that's super stretchy or fragile

- Easy bruising and poor wound healing
- Organ prolapse (yeah, it's as fun as it sounds)
- Chronic pain from unstable joints

But here's where it connects to MCAS: connective tissue is everywhere, including around your mast cells. Abnormal connective tissue might affect how mast cells behave. Plus, the chronic inflammation from MCAS can further damage already fragile connective tissue. It's a vicious cycle.

POTS - When Standing Up Becomes an Olympic Sport

POTS means your heart rate jumps by 30+ beats per minute (or over 120) when you stand up. But it's not just a heart thing. Symptoms include:

- Dizziness or fainting upon standing
- Brain fog that worsens upright
- Fatigue that's positional
- Nausea and GI issues
- Temperature regulation problems

Sound familiar? Many POTS symptoms overlap with MCAS. That's because mast cells release chemicals that affect blood vessels and heart rate. Some researchers think MCAS might actually cause POTS in some people (Shibao et al., 2005).

The Connection Game

So why do these three show up together? Several theories:

1. **Genetic factors**: Some genetic mutations might predispose to all three
2. **Structural issues**: Loose connective tissue affects mast cell behavior
3. **Inflammatory cascade**: Each condition triggers inflammation that worsens the others

105

4. **Nervous system dysfunction**: All three involve autonomic nervous system problems

Jessica (fictional name, real pattern) had joint pain for years. Doctors said she was "just flexible." Then came the digestive issues, diagnosed as IBS. When she started fainting, she got a POTS diagnosis. It took five more years before someone connected the dots to MCAS. Treating the MCAS improved all her other symptoms. The conditions were talking to each other all along.

Long COVID: The New Kid on the Block

Then came 2020, and suddenly millions of people developed multi-system symptoms that looked suspiciously like... MCAS. Long COVID symptoms include:

- Fatigue that doesn't match exertion
- Brain fog and cognitive issues
- Heart palpitations and chest pain
- Shortness of breath
- GI problems
- Skin rashes
- Temperature dysregulation

Researchers found that COVID can trigger mast cell activation, and this might explain many long COVID symptoms (Weinstock et al., 2021). For people with pre-existing MCAS, COVID can be like pouring gasoline on a fire. For others, COVID might be the trigger that activates previously quiet mast cells.

The Long COVID-MCAS Connection

Several mechanisms might explain this connection:

- Viral particles directly triggering mast cells

- Immune system overreaction leading to persistent activation
- Damage to tissues that normally keep mast cells in check
- Autoimmune responses affecting mast cell regulation

If you developed weird multi-system symptoms after COVID that won't go away, MCAS should be on your radar. The good news? MCAS treatments often help long COVID symptoms, even if we don't fully understand why yet.

Autoimmune Overlaps

MCAS also plays well (or poorly) with autoimmune conditions:

Hashimoto's Thyroiditis

- Mast cells infiltrate the thyroid
- Inflammation affects hormone production
- Symptoms overlap (fatigue, brain fog, temperature issues)

Rheumatoid Arthritis

- Mast cells contribute to joint inflammation
- RA treatments might worsen MCAS
- Flares often coincide

Lupus

- Both involve inappropriate immune activation
- Photosensitivity common in both
- Inflammatory cascades interact

Multiple Sclerosis

- Mast cells found in MS lesions
- Both have neurological symptoms

- Stress triggers both conditions

The connection? Mast cells are part of your immune system. When they're overactive, they can trigger or worsen autoimmune responses. Plus, the inflammation from autoimmune conditions can further activate mast cells.

The Gut Connection: When IBS Isn't Just IBS

How many people get diagnosed with IBS when they actually have MCAS? We don't know exact numbers, but it's probably a lot. Consider that mast cells:

- Are abundant in the gut lining
- React to foods and stress
- Cause cramping, diarrhea, and bloating
- Create inflammation that mimics IBS

Studies show increased mast cells in IBS patients' intestines (Barbara et al., 2004). Some researchers argue that certain IBS cases are actually localized mast cell activation. If your "IBS" comes with flushing, itching, or other systemic symptoms, consider MCAS.

Fibromyalgia: Another Misunderstood Connection

Fibromyalgia's widespread pain, fatigue, and cognitive issues overlap significantly with MCAS. Some researchers found increased mast cells in fibromyalgia patients' skin (Blanco et al., 2010). The pain might result from mast cell mediators affecting nerve endings.

Signs your fibromyalgia might involve mast cells:

- Pain that comes with flushing or rashes
- Symptoms triggered by foods or environmental factors
- Improvement with antihistamines

- Multiple chemical sensitivities

Creating Your Personal Diagnostic Map

Understanding your condition constellation helps target treatment. Here's a flowchart approach:

Start with your primary symptoms:

If joint hypermobility + chronic pain → Evaluate for EDS ↓ If also have POTS symptoms → Check standing heart rate ↓ If multiple triggers cause reactions → Consider MCAS evaluation

If chronic fatigue + multi-system symptoms → Consider:

- Post-viral syndromes (including long COVID)
- Autoimmune conditions
- MCAS as underlying factor

If diagnosed with IBS/fibromyalgia but treatments aren't helping → Look for:

- Triggers beyond stress
- Skin symptoms
- Response to antihistamines
- Family history of allergies/sensitivities

The Diagnostic Journey: Connecting the Dots

Getting diagnosed with one condition often leads to discovering others. The key is finding doctors who understand these connections.

Red flags that suggest multiple conditions:

- Symptoms affecting 3+ body systems
- Onset after infection or major stress

- Family history of hypermobility or allergies
- Partial response to single-condition treatments
- Symptoms that seem unrelated but flare together

Treatment Implications

Understanding comorbidities changes treatment approaches:

Integrated Treatment Planning:

- Address the most fundamental condition first (often MCAS)
- Watch for medication interactions
- Coordinate between specialists
- Track which treatments help multiple conditions

Medication Considerations:

- Some medications help multiple conditions (win!)
- Others might worsen comorbidities (careful!)
- Start low and go slow
- Monitor all symptoms, not just target ones

Lifestyle Modifications:

- Changes that help one condition often help others
- Stress management benefits everything
- Diet modifications might address multiple issues
- Exercise needs careful planning with multiple conditions

Success Stories: The Power of Connection

Let me tell you about David (fictional name, real results). He had:

- Chronic fatigue diagnosed as depression
- Joint pain attributed to "getting older" (at 35!)

- Heart palpitations labeled as anxiety
- Digestive issues diagnosed as IBS

Four specialists. Four separate treatments. Minimal improvement.

Then he saw an immunologist who recognized the pattern. Testing revealed MCAS, with secondary POTS and hypermobile joints suggesting EDS. Starting MCAS treatment improved everything:

- Fatigue lifted significantly
- Joint pain decreased
- Heart palpitations nearly resolved
- Digestive issues became manageable

The conditions weren't separate problems. They were different manifestations of the same underlying dysfunction.

The Family Connection

These conditions often run in families, though they might manifest differently:

- Mom has "allergies" and migraines
- Sister has endometriosis and anxiety
- Brother has IBS and eczema
- Child has growing pains and food sensitivities

Looking at family patterns helps identify genetic predispositions and guide early intervention.

Moving Forward with Multiple Conditions

Living with multiple conditions requires strategy:

1. **Find an anchor doctor** who understands the connections
2. **Keep comprehensive records** accessible to all providers
3. **Track symptoms holistically**, not by condition
4. **Advocate for integrated care** rather than siloed treatment
5. **Connect with others** who have similar combinations
6. **Celebrate small wins** - improving one condition often helps others

The Research Horizon

Researchers are finally recognizing these connections. Current studies explore:

- Genetic markers linking conditions
- Shared inflammatory pathways
- Integrated treatment protocols
- Early identification strategies

As understanding grows, diagnosis and treatment will improve. You're not crazy for thinking your conditions are connected. They probably are.

Building Your Healthcare Team

With multiple conditions, you need:

- A primary care doctor who sees the big picture
- Specialists who communicate with each other
- Providers willing to think outside their specialty box
- Support professionals (PT, therapy, nutrition)

The Hope Factor

Having multiple conditions sounds overwhelming, but there's hope:

- Understanding connections leads to better treatment
- Addressing root causes improves multiple symptoms
- You're not alone - many share your combination
- Research is advancing rapidly
- Integrated treatment works

The goal isn't to cure everything overnight. It's to understand how your body's systems interact and use that knowledge to feel better. Every piece of the puzzle you identify brings you closer to effective management.

Key Takeaways

- MCAS rarely occurs alone - it often appears with EDS, POTS, and autoimmune conditions
- These conditions share inflammatory pathways and may have common genetic factors
- Long COVID can trigger or unmask MCAS in previously healthy people
- Many IBS and fibromyalgia cases may actually involve mast cell activation
- Understanding condition connections leads to more effective treatment
- Family patterns provide clues to genetic predispositions
- Integrated treatment addressing root causes improves multiple conditions
- Building a knowledgeable healthcare team is crucial
- Research is advancing rapidly, offering hope for better diagnosis and treatment

Chapter 11: Living with MCAS – Patient Stories and Coping

Life with MCAS isn't just about managing symptoms. It's about rebuilding your entire existence around a body that seems to have declared war on the modern world. It's about explaining to your boss why fluorescent lights make you sick, or telling your date that you need to check every ingredient in the restaurant's kitchen. It's about feeling like an alien in your own life while trying to maintain some semblance of normalcy.

But here's what the medical journals don't tell you: people with MCAS aren't just surviving. They're living, loving, working, and thriving. Sure, it takes creativity, planning, and more backup plans than a NASA mission. But it's possible. And sometimes, the journey of learning to live with MCAS teaches you things about resilience you never knew you had.

Sarah's Story: From Mystery to Mastery

Sarah was 28 when her body started rebelling. A successful marketing manager, she prided herself on juggling multiple projects while training for marathons. Then came the hives during a client dinner. "I thought it was shellfish," she told me. "Stopped eating seafood. But the reactions kept coming."

Within six months, Sarah's world had shrunk. Wine with friends triggered flushing and rapid heartbeat. Her morning runs caused widespread itching. Perfume in the office made her throat feel tight. "I became that person," she said. "The one with the weird food restrictions and strange requests. I felt like a burden everywhere I went."

The medical odyssey began. Allergists found no IgE allergies. Cardiologists said her heart was fine. Dermatologists prescribed creams that didn't help. A psychiatrist suggested anxiety medication. "I started doubting myself. Maybe I was going crazy. Maybe I was making it all up for attention."

Year three brought a new allergist who'd recently attended an MCAS conference. He listened to Sarah's full story - the seemingly random reactions, the exercise intolerance, the way stress made everything worse. Labs during a reaction showed elevated prostaglandins. Finally, a diagnosis.

"I cried," Sarah admitted. "Not because I was sick, but because I wasn't crazy. There was a real, biological reason for what was happening."

Treatment wasn't instant magic. H1 and H2 blockers helped but caused drowsiness. Cromolyn made things worse before better. Finding her trigger patterns took months of meticulous tracking. But slowly, life expanded again.

Today, Sarah still has MCAS. But she also has a modified marathon schedule (early morning, cool weather only), a fragrance-free workspace, and a restaurant list where she can eat safely. "I can't do everything I used to," she said. "But I can do more than I thought I'd ever do again. And I appreciate it all so much more."

Michael's Journey: When MCAS Hits in Midlife

Michael was 45, married with two teenagers, when long COVID changed everything. The acute infection was mild. The aftermath wasn't. "Three months after recovery, I was sicker than during the actual COVID," he explained.

Fatigue that felt like wearing a lead suit. Brain fog that made his engineering work impossible. Rashes that appeared from

115

nowhere. Stomach cramps after every meal. His wife Emma watched him transform from family rock to someone who could barely leave bed.

"The hardest part was my kids seeing me like that," Michael said. "My son had to help me up the stairs. My daughter was afraid to hug me because she might trigger a reaction."

Multiple doctors, multiple theories. Chronic fatigue syndrome. Depression. Anxiety. Deconditioning. "One doctor actually said I should try harder to exercise. I couldn't walk to the mailbox without collapsing, and he wanted me to try harder?"

A long COVID clinic finally connected the dots. Michael's symptoms fit MCAS triggered by viral infection. Treatment started conservatively - antihistamines, mast cell stabilizers, dietary changes. Progress was glacial but real.

"The first time I made it through dinner without running to the bathroom, Emma cried," he remembered. "Such a small thing, but it meant maybe we'd get our life back."

Michael's not back to his pre-COVID self. He works part-time from home. Exercise means gentle walks, not mountain biking. The family adapted - fragrance-free everything, HEPA filters throughout the house, backup plans for every outing.

"My kids joke that I'm bionic now - all these supplements and medications keeping me running," he laughed. "But they also understand chronic illness in a way I wish they didn't have to. They're more compassionate people because of it."

Emma's Experience: The Pediatric MCAS Journey

Emma (different Emma) was just 8 when the stomach aches started. Her mom, Lisa, initially blamed school anxiety. But then came the rashes, the sudden food aversions, the times Emma would flush bright red for no reason.

"Doctors kept saying she'd outgrow it," Lisa recalled. "Growing pains. Childhood anxieties. One suggested she was seeking attention because her younger brother was born. I knew something was really wrong, but nobody listened to the mom."

The breaking point came during a school field trip. Emma had a severe reaction - hives, vomiting, difficulty breathing. The ER gave Benadryl and sent them home with an EpiPen "just in case." But Lisa demanded answers.

Finding a pediatric MCAS specialist took six months and required traveling two states away. The diagnosis brought relief and terror. "How do you explain to an 8-year-old that her body is allergic to life?" Lisa wondered.

Treatment for pediatric MCAS requires extra creativity. Emma couldn't swallow pills, so medications were compounded into liquids. Dietary restrictions had to account for growth needs. School required extensive accommodation plans.

"The hardest part is the social aspect," Lisa explained. "Birthday parties with food she can't eat. Sleepovers where everything has fragrance. Kids don't understand why Emma can't just have one bite of cake."

But kids are also remarkably adaptable. Emma learned to advocate for herself. She carries safe snacks everywhere. She knows which friends' houses are safe. She matter-of-factly explains her condition to curious classmates.

"Sometimes I feel guilty," Lisa admitted. "Other parents worry about screen time. I worry about anaphylaxis. But Emma is thriving in her own way. She's resilient, empathetic, and wise beyond her years. MCAS is part of her story, not her whole story."

The Emotional Rollercoaster

Living with MCAS means riding waves of emotions:

Grief for the life you planned **Anger** at your body's betrayal **Fear** of reactions and the future **Isolation** from a world that doesn't understand **Hope** when treatments work **Joy** in small victories **Frustration** with setbacks **Gratitude** for good days

These feelings aren't sequential stages. They're recurring visitors, showing up unexpectedly. Tuesday's hope becomes Wednesday's despair. Friday's confidence crumbles with Saturday's reaction. And that's okay. That's normal. That's human.

Explaining the Unexplainable

How do you explain MCAS to people who've never heard of it?

The Short Version: "I have a condition where my immune system overreacts to normal things. Think of it like having allergies to life itself."

The Medium Version: "My mast cells - part of my immune system - release chemicals inappropriately. This causes reactions that look like allergies but aren't. I have to avoid certain triggers and take medications to stay stable."

The Detailed Version (for those who genuinely want to understand): Explain mast cells, mediators, triggers, and why reactions seem random. Use analogies they can relate to.

For Employers: Focus on accommodations needed and your ability to work with them. Provide medical documentation. Emphasize solutions, not just problems.

For Friends and Family: Be honest about limitations but also about possibilities. Help them understand how they can support you.

Dealing with Doubters

Not everyone will believe or understand. Common responses and how to handle them:

"But you don't look sick" → "Many chronic illnesses are invisible. I'm good at managing my symptoms, but they're still there."

"Have you tried yoga/supplements/positive thinking?" → "I appreciate your concern. I'm working with doctors on a treatment plan that's helping."

"It's all in your head" → "MCAS is a recognized medical condition with biological markers. I'd be happy to share some information if you're interested."

"You're too focused on being sick" → "I focus on it exactly as much as needed to stay functional. Trust me, I'd rather think about anything else."

Building Your Support Network

Isolation makes everything worse. Building connection helps:

Online Communities:

- The Mast Cell Disease Society forums

119

- Facebook groups (choose carefully - some are more helpful than others)
- Reddit r/MCAS community
- Instagram accounts sharing MCAS experiences

Local Support:

- Rare disease support groups
- Chronic illness meetups
- MCAS-aware healthcare providers who can connect patients

Creating Boundaries:

- It's okay to limit time with people who drain your energy
- You don't owe everyone a detailed explanation
- "No" is a complete sentence
- Your health comes before social obligations

Practical Coping Strategies

The Emergency Kit Philosophy: Always have:

- Medications (daily and rescue)
- Safe snacks
- Water
- Medical information card
- Comfort items (sunglasses, earplugs, whatever helps)

The Three-Plan Rule: Plan A: The ideal scenario Plan B: The backup Plan C: The escape route

Energy Budgeting:

- Treat energy like money - limited supply
- Prioritize essential activities
- Bank energy before big events

- Plan recovery time
- Learn to delegate

Creating Safe Spaces:

- Make your bedroom a trigger-free sanctuary
- Have one safe restaurant you can always count on
- Identify friends' homes where you can relax
- Know which stores/locations are generally safe

Working with MCAS

Employment brings unique challenges:

Disclosure Decisions:

- You're not required to disclose unless requesting accommodations
- Focus on abilities and solutions
- Provide specific accommodation requests
- Get everything in writing

Common Accommodations:

- Fragrance-free workspace
- Flexible scheduling for medical appointments
- Work-from-home options
- Temperature control access
- Break time for medications

Career Pivots: Some people change careers to better accommodate MCAS:

- Remote work opportunities
- Self-employment for ultimate control
- Part-time or freelance arrangements
- Industries with fewer triggers

Parenting with MCAS

Being a parent with MCAS requires extra planning:

- Explain your condition age-appropriately
- Involve kids in safe meal planning
- Have backup caregivers for flare days
- Create fun within limitations
- Model good self-care

When Your Child Has MCAS:

- Educate teachers and caregivers thoroughly
- Create detailed care plans
- Teach self-advocacy early
- Connect with other MCAS families
- Celebrate their resilience

Finding Joy Despite MCAS

Life with MCAS isn't all restrictions and reactions. People find joy in:

- Deeper connections with understanding friends
- Appreciation for good days
- Creative problem-solving skills
- New hobbies that fit limitations
- Helping others with similar struggles
- Simple pleasures previously taken for granted

The Growth Through Struggle

Many people with MCAS report unexpected personal growth:

- Increased empathy for others' invisible struggles
- Better boundaries and self-advocacy
- Clarity about what truly matters

- Resilience they didn't know they had
- Deeper spiritual or philosophical perspectives
- Stronger genuine relationships

Resources for Your Journey

Organizations:

- The Mastocytosis Society: tmsforacure.org
- Mast Cell Action: mastcellaction.org
- MCAS Hope: mcashope.com

Finding Specialists:

- TMS physician database
- MCAS Hope provider list
- Local university medical centers
- Functional medicine practitioners with MCAS experience

Educational Resources:

- "Never Bet Against Occam" by Dr. Lawrence Afrin
- MCAS research updates on PubMed
- Reputable MCAS blogs and podcasts
- Medical conference videos online

Practical Tools:

- Symptom tracking apps
- Medical ID bracelets
- Medication reminder systems
- Air quality monitors
- Safe product databases

A Message of Hope

If you're newly diagnosed, drowning in symptoms, or feeling hopeless, hear this: It gets better. Not perfect. Not cured. But better. You'll learn your triggers. You'll find treatments that help. You'll discover a strength you didn't know existed.

You'll also find your people - others who understand the bizarre reality of reacting to seemingly everything. Who get why you carry Benadryl like a lifeline. Who celebrate with you when you tolerate a new food or make it through an event reaction-free.

MCAS changes your life, no question. But it doesn't end it. People with MCAS are traveling (carefully), working (creatively), loving (deeply), and living (fully). Your journey will be unique, with its own challenges and victories.

The path forward isn't about returning to who you were before MCAS. It's about becoming who you're meant to be with it - likely more compassionate, resilient, and grateful than you ever imagined possible. And that person? They're worth fighting for.

Key Takeaways

- MCAS affects entire families and requires adjustment from everyone
- Patient stories show that improvement is possible with proper treatment and lifestyle changes
- Emotional responses to chronic illness are normal and recurring
- Building a support network is crucial for managing MCAS
- Practical strategies like emergency kits and energy budgeting improve daily life
- Work accommodations can enable continued employment
- Children with MCAS can thrive with proper support and advocacy
- Finding joy and meaning is possible despite limitations

- Personal growth often emerges from the struggle
- Resources and community support are available
- Hope is justified - life with MCAS can be full and meaningful

Reference

- Abraham, S. N., & St John, A. L. (2010). Mast cell–orchestrated immunity to pathogens. *Nature Reviews Immunology, 10*(6), 440–452.

- Afrin, L. B. (2013). Presentation, diagnosis, and management of mast cell activation syndrome. In *Mast Cells* (pp. 155–232). Nova Science Publishers.

- Afrin, L. B., Butterfield, J. H., Raithel, M., & Molderings, G. J. (2016). Often seen, rarely recognized: Mast cell activation disease—a guide to diagnosis and therapeutic options. *Annals of Medicine, 48*(3), 190–201.

- Barbara, G., Stanghellini, V., De Giorgio, R., Cremon, C., Cottrell, G. S., Santini, D., ... & Corinaldesi, R. (2004). Activated mast cells in proximity to colonic nerves correlate with abdominal pain in irritable bowel syndrome. *Gastroenterology, 126*(3), 693–702.

- Blanco, I., Béritze, N., Argüelles, M., Cárcaba, V., Fernández, F., Janciauskiene, S., ... & Astudillo, A. (2010). Abnormal overexpression of mastocytes in skin biopsies of fibromyalgia patients. *Clinical Rheumatology, 29*(12), 1403–1412.

- Cheung, I., & Vadas, P. (2015). A new disease cluster: Mast cell activation syndrome, postural orthostatic tachycardia syndrome, and Ehlers–Danlos syndrome [Abstract]. *Journal of Allergy and Clinical Immunology, 135*(2), AB65.

- Hamilton, M. J., Hornick, J. L., Akin, C., Castells, M. C., & Greenberger, N. J. (2011). Mast cell activation syndrome: A newly recognized disorder with systemic clinical manifestations. *Journal of Allergy and Clinical Immunology, 128*(1), 147–152.

- Krystel-Whittemore, M., Dileepan, K. N., & Wood, J. G. (2016). Mast cell: A multi-functional master cell. *Frontiers in Immunology, 6,* 620.

- Lyons, J. J. (2018). Hereditary alpha tryptasemia: Genotyping and associated clinical features. *Immunology and Allergy Clinics of North America, 38*(3), 483–495.

- Lyons, J. J., Yu, X., Hughes, J. D., Le, Q. T., Jamil, A., Bai, Y., ... & Milner, J. D. (2016). Elevated basal serum tryptase identifies a multisystem disorder associated with increased *TPSAB1* copy number. *Nature Genetics, 48*(12), 1564–1569.

- Maintz, L., & Novak, N. (2007). Histamine and histamine intolerance. *The American Journal of Clinical Nutrition, 85*(5), 1185–1196.

- Maintz, L., Yu, C. F., Rodríguez, E., Baurecht, H., Bieber, T., Illig, T., ... & Novak, N. (2011). Association of single nucleotide polymorphisms in the diamine oxidase gene with diamine oxidase serum activities. *Allergy, 66*(7), 893–902.

- Molderings, G. J., Brettner, S., Homann, J., & Afrin, L. B. (2011). Mast cell activation disease: A concise practical guide for diagnostic workup and therapeutic options. *Journal of Hematology & Oncology, 4,* 10.

- Schnedl, W. J., & Enko, D. (2021). Histamine intolerance originates in the gut. *Nutrients, 13*(4), 1262.

- Schnedl, W. J., Lackner, S., Enko, D., Schenk, M., Holasek, S. J., & Mangge, H. (2019). Evaluation of symptoms and symptom combinations in histamine intolerance. *Intestinal Research, 17*(3), 427–433.

- Shibao, C., Arzubiaga, C., Roberts, L. J., Raj, S., Black, B., Harris, P., & Biaggioni, I. (2005). Hyperadrenergic postural tachycardia syndrome in mast cell activation disorders. *Hypertension, 45*(3), 385–390.

- Theoharides, T. C., & Kavalioti, M. (2018). Stress, inflammation and natural treatments. *Journal of Biological Regulators & Homeostatic Agents(editorial).*

- Theoharides, T. C., Alysandratos, K. D., Angelidou, A., Delivanis, D. A., Sismanopoulos, N., Zhang, B., ... & Kalogeromitros, D. (2012). Mast cells and inflammation. *Biochimica et Biophysica Acta (BBA) – Molecular Basis of Disease, 1822*(1), 21–33.

- Theoharides, T. C., Stewart, J. M., Hatziagelaki, E., & Kolaitis, G. (2015). Brain "fog," inflammation and obesity: Key aspects of neuropsychiatric disorders improved by luteolin. *Frontiers in Neuroscience, 9,* 225.

- Valent, P., Akin, C., Arock, M., Brockow, K., Butterfield, J. H., Carter, M. C., ... & Metcalfe, D. D. (2012). Definitions, criteria and global classification of mast cell disorders with special reference to mast cell activation syndromes: A consensus proposal.

International Archives of Allergy and Immunology,
157(3), 215–225.

- Weinstock, L. B., Brook, J. B., Walters, A. S., Goris, A.,
  Afrin, L. B., & Molderings, G. J. (2021). Mast cell
  activation symptoms are prevalent in long-COVID.
  International Journal of Infectious Diseases, 112,
  217–226.